Resolution, Properties, and Genetic Aspects of Complement

Volume I in MSS' Series on Complement

Papers by
Kunio Yonemasu, Carlos R. Sledge, David H. Bing et al.

MSS Information Corporation
655 Madison Avenue, New York, N.Y. 10021

Library of Congress Cataloging in Publication Data

Main entry under title:

Resolution, properties, and genetic aspects of
    complement.

    (MSS' Series on complement, v. 1)
    1. Complements (Immunity)--Addresses, essays,
Lectures. I. Yonemasu, Kunio. II. Sledge, Carlos R.
III. Bing, David H. IV: Series. [DNLM: 1. Complement
Collected works. QW680 R434 1974]
QR185.8.C6M17 Vol. 1   599'.02'9s [599'.02'9]
ISBN 0-8422-7229-1   74-8406

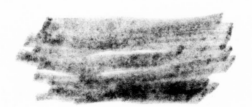

TABLE OF CONTENTS

CREDITS AND ACKNOWLEDGEMENTS

Agnello, V.; M.M.E. de Bracco; and H.G. Kunkel, "Hereditary C2 Deficiency with Some Manifestations of Systemic Lupus Erythematosus," *The Journal of Immunology*, 1972, 108:837-840.

Arroyave, Carlos M.; and Hans J. Müller-Eberhard, "Isolation of the Sixth Component of Complement from Human Serum," *Immunochemistry*, 1971, 8:995-1006.

Bing, David H., "Purification of the Human Complement Protein Cls̄ by Affinity Chromatography," *Immunochemistry*, 1971, 8:539-550.

Colten, Harvey R.; and Chester A. Alper, "Hemolytic Efficiencies of Genetic Variants of Human C3," *The Journal of Immunology*, 1972, 108:1184-1187.

Colten, H.R.; and M.M. Frank, "Biosynthesis of the Second (C2) and Fourth (C4) Components of Complement *in Vitro* by Tissues Isolated from Guinea-Pigs with Genetically Determined C4 Deficiency," *Immunology*, 1972, 22:991-999.

Nilsson, U.R.; R.H. Tomar; and F.B. Taylor, Jr., "Additional Studies on Human C5: Development of a Modified Purification Method and Characterization of the Purified Product by Polyacrylamide Gel Electrophoresis," *Immunochemistry*, 1972, 9:709-723.

Sassano, Felix G.; Harvey R. Colten; Tibor Borsos; and Herbert J. Rapp, "Resolution of the First Complement of Guinea Pig Complement into Three Subunits, Clg, Clr and Cls, and Their Hybridization with Human Cl Subunits," *Immunochemistry*, 1972, 9:405-412.

Shelton, Emma; Kunio Yonemasu; and Robert M. Stroud, "Ultrastructure of the Human Complement Component, Clq," *Proceedings of the National Academy of Sciences*, 1972, 69:65-68.

Sledge, Carlos R.; and David H. Bing, "Purification of the Human Complement Protein Clq by Affinity Chromatography," *The Journal of Immunology*, 1973, 3:661-666.

Thompson, James J.; and Louis G. Hoffmann, "Function and Physical Properties of Two Distinct Forms of the First Component of Guinea Pig Complement," *Immunochemistry*, 1971, 8:169-184.

Yonemasu, Kunio; and Robert M. Stroud, "Clq: Rapid Purification Method for Preparation of Monospecific Antisera and for Biochemical Studies," *The Journal of Immunology*, 1971, 106:304-313.

Yonemasu, Kunio; and Robert M. Stroud, "Structural Studies on Human Clq: Non-Covalent and Covalent Subunits," *Immunochemistry*, 1972, 9:545-554.

Yonemasu, Kunio; Robert M. Stroud; William Niedermeier; and William T. Butler, "Chemical Studies on Clq: A Modulator of Immunoglobulin Biology," *Biochemical and Biophysical Research Communications*, 1971, 43:1388-1394.

PREFACE

Complement may generally be described as a complex system of eleven distinct serum proteins which interacts through various mechanisms with the antibody portion of immune complexes and cellular components to preserve the delicate balance between health and disease in the organism.

Although the earliest reference to complement activity in serum has been traced to 1895, little was known about the structure, other physical and chemical properties or the molecular mechanisms of action until relatively recently. A small number of dedicated research groups around the world have diligently sought to understand and describe complement during the last two decades. A committee, sponsored by the World Health Organization, even defined the symbols and acceptable nomenclature of this complex biological system in 1970 (see Yonemasu). In addition, numerous International immunologic congresses and symposia have been held in the past five years with complement as the sole topic.

A crucial pre-requisite for understanding the specific mechanism of action in any biological system is knowing the composition of the moieties and catalysts. During the last fifteen years, purification methods have been devised which allow for the separation of each of the component units of complement. Owing to the beta globulin-like behavior of these proteins, — they all have similar electrophoretic mobility, — sophisticated techniques were required to determine that there were eleven protein units. Batch preparation of enough of each of the proteins to do functional and structural studies often required the development of additional procedures.

This volume, the first in a series on complement, contains a number of articles on the isolation and purification of various proteins of complement. The techniques used in these endeavors include multiple precipitations with chelating agents, affinity chromatography and ultracentrifugation in sucrose gradients. Resolution of each of the eleven component units requires special techniques which recognize the relatively minor unique physical and chemical features of each protein to separate it from the other ten. Certain contaminants are described which tend to de-activate the proteins; techniques for the removal of such de-activators are described when known. Standard characterization of the purified product is routinely made by gel electrophoresis; biological activity is described in many reports. Polyacrylamide gel electrophoresis at alkaline pH allows for the migration of all eleven component proteins, once relatively uncontaminated, into unique bands.

The molecular weights have been determined to range from 400,000 for C1q to 80,000 for both C1s and C9. Descriptions of studies are included in which highly resolved components of complement are hybridized and reactivated.

Functional and physical property studies of complement have only been possible since large quantities of purified complement components were obtainable. Volume II of this series contains a series of reports on the action of complement in the biological system. The ultrastructural studies included in this volume indicate that at least the C1q component is a fragile molecule of three distinct parts. Knowledge regarding the structure of the various units and their physical relationship to each other is providing clues to the function of complement in its various specific roles.

As might be expected from any complex system that plays such a significant part in body processes, the absence of or any aberrations in the structure of the complement components or in their initiating enzymes produces an abnormal state which is likely to adversely affect the individual. A few articles on genetically related complement deficiencies are included in this selection.

Ronald T. Acton, Ph.D.
June, 1974

Resolution

Clq: RAPID PURIFICATION METHOD FOR PREPARATION OF MONOSPECIFIC ANTISERA AND FOR BIOCHEMICAL STUDIES[1,2]

KUNIO YONEMASU AND ROBERT M. STROUD

Clq has been purified using precipitation in the presence of chelating agents at low ionic strength. The three times precipitated Clq was highly purified as shown by immunoelectrophoresis and analytic acrylamide disc electrophoresis. On immunoelectrophoresis, the purified Clq showed a single line in the slow λ-region against a potent anti-whole human anti-serum, and the hemolytic activity and latex agglutination activity of Clq coincided with this region.

The final product showed hemolytic activity and latex agglutination activity but did not show any detectable Clr or Cls activity. The yield of Clq using these methods is about 40 to 60% and thus about 5 mg can be obtained from 100 ml of serum. The highly purified Clq obtained from 3.75% preparative acrylamide gels containing sodium dodecyl sulfate yields potent monospecific antisera when injected into rabbits. These antisera agglutinate EAClq cells but not EA. The molecular weight of Clq as estimated by its relative mobility on acrylamide gels was 387,600 ± 10,790, and breakdown to smaller subunits has been demonstrated in gels containing urea.

[1] This work was supported by grants from the National Institutes of Health, United States Public Health Service, and from the Veterans Administration.

[2] The symbols for complement components used in this paper conform to the recommendations of a committee sponsored by the World Health Organization. "Nomenclature of Complement," Immunochemistry, 7: 137, 1970. Complement (C) components are designated numerically C1, C2, C3, C4, C5, C6, C7, C8 and C9; the subunits of C1 are designated Clq, Clr and Cls; activated components are indicated by placing a bar over the numeral which refers to the component or subunit, i.e., active C1 = C$\bar{1}$; active Cls = C$\bar{1}$s. As guinea pig components are always used for the C1 subunits which were from human serum, a superscript indicating the species will be omitted. Cellular intermediates carrying C components are designated EAC, followed by the numeral designating the components carried, e.g., EAC$\bar{1}$4.

The first component of human complement, C1, is known to consist of three subunits, C1q, C1r and C1s, whose function as a unit requires Ca^{++} (1). C1q was originally isolated by Müller-Eberhard and Kunkel (2), who described the ability of this heat-labile protein to interact with and to precipitate γ globulins from solutions in the presence of EDTA. This purified 11S protein reconstituted the diminished complement activity in whole serum which had been depleted of C1q. Precipitation of antigen-antibody complexes was previously described to be a function of a heat-labile complement component in experiments by Weigle and Maurer (3), and the increased insolubility of antigen-antibody complexes or denatured IgG has been confirmed in agar diffusion experiments (4, 5). The initial binding site between complement protein and antigen-antibody complexes is considered to be on C1q. When C1q is combined with its subunits in the presence of Ca^{++}, the complement sequence is initiated by activation of C1s (6). C1q is not thought to have an enzymatic function in contradistinction to C1r and C1s. The initial stimulus for C1s activation after C1 is bound is probably an allosteric effect allowing C1r to enzymatically activate C1s (7); however, further study is required. Certain classes of IgG (8) and IgM (9) do not bind C1q. A weak reversible binding of C1q to monomers of certain IgG subclasses has been demonstrated (8). If binding data on C1 are applicable to C1q, firm binding appears to require a doublet of IgG molecules (10), but higher order immunoglobulin polymers contribute to the binding strength (11). On the other hand, a single IgM molecule will bind a single C1 molecule (10), perhaps because of cooperative effects between the five 7S subunits. Hyslop *et al.* (12) have recently suggested that the bond angle between the two arms of the Fab portion of IgG is of significance in this binding. Müller-Eberhard has reported that C1q is multivalent for IgG. A maximal estimate of five IgG molecules is bound for every C1q molecule. The binding site appears to be on the invariant portion of the H chain (13).

A method of purification has been outlined by Müller-Eberhard (8), but in our hands this method gave low yields. Purified C1q is important for the production of monospecific antisera for clinical studies. Furthermore, functionally intact C1q is of increasing clinical importance for detection of soluble altered immunoglobulins or antigen-antibody complexes (14). Improved purification yields will facilitate structural studies. The method presented here is an improved method for purification, and it should have widespread use. Data on purification yields, preparation of monospecific antisera and selected biochemical studies are presented.

Source of human C1q. Normal human blood was clotted at room temperature for 60 min and then allowed to retract at 0°C for 120 min. Serum was separated by centrifugation at 0 to 4°C and recentrifuged at 20,000 $\times$ G for 90 min in order to aspirate free lipid.

Complement components. Pooled guinea pig serum was purchased from Texas Biologicals, Inc., Fort Worth, Texas. Functionally pure guinea pig C2 was prepared using the method of Nelson *et al.* (15). C-EDTA was made by diluting guinea pig serum 1:50 with EDTA buffer. Human C1r and C1s were purified and assayed according to described methods (16, 17).

Cellular intermediates. E, EA and EAC$\bar{1}$4 were prepared as described by Mayer (18). EAC4 cells were prepared according to Borsos and Rapp (19).

Buffers. The RSC (relative salt concentration) refers to a solution of NaCl giving the same electrical resistance at 0°C. Isotonic Veronal-buffered saline (VBS) (RSC = 0.147, pH 7.4) was prepared according to Mayer (18). Veronal-buffered dextrose saline (DGVB^{++}), (RSC = 0.075, pH 7.4; and RSC = 0.065, pH 7.4) was prepared by mixing isotonic Veronal-buffered saline with 5% dextrose to the desired RSC. These buffers contained MgCl$_2$, CaCl$_2$ and gelatin to a final concentration of 1 mM, 0.15 mM and 0.1%, respectively. EDTA buffer was prepared by making a 1:10 dilution of stock 0.1 M trisodium ethylenediamine tetraacetate (pH 7.4) with VBS. EDTA-Veronal-buffered dextrose (EDTA-DGVB) (RSC = 0.065, pH 7.4) was prepared by mixing EDTA buffer with 5% dextrose containing 0.1% gelatin to yield the desired resistance.

Reagents. Ethyleneglycol bis (aminoethyl)-tetraacetic acid (EGTA) and EDTA were puchased from the G. Frederick Smith Chemical Co., Columbus, Ohio, and Eastman Organic Chemicals, Rochester, N. Y., respectively, and the solutions used for purification were adjusted by measuring the electrical resistance (RSC). Sodium dodecyl sulfate (SDS) was purchased from K & K Laboratories, Plainview, N. Y. Agarose (lot 381217) was purchased from Bausch & Lomb Optical Co., Rochester, N. Y. Bacto-Latex was purchased from Difco Laboratories, Detroit, Mich. Gamma globulin as fraction II was a gift from Merck Sharp & Dohme Research Laboratories, West Point, Pa. A certified ammonium sulfate nitrogen standard and Nessler's reagent (Koch-McMeekin) were purchased from Sargent Laboratories, Birmingham, Ala. Crystalline human serum albumin dried *in vacuo* to a constant weight was also used as a nitrogen standard. Horse antibody to whole human serum was obtained from Microbial Diseases Research Foundation, Osaka University.

Immunodiffusion analysis. a) Ouchterlony double diffusion was carried out in 1% agarose in 0.05 M Tris and 0.05 M glycine-buffered 0.15 M NaCl containing 0.01 M EDTA and 0.1% Na-azide, RSC = 0.18, pH 8.0, as supporting medium. b) Immunoelectrophoresis was carried out according to a modification of the method of Scheidegger (20) using 1% agarose in Veronal-acetate buffer containing 0.01 M EDTA. c) Radial immunodiffusion (RID) was carried out according to a modification of Mancini *et al.* (21) with 1% agarose containing a proper dilution of rabbit antibody to C1q in the buffered saline used for Ouchterlony analysis. For quantitative assay of human IgG or IgM immunoplates containing antihuman IgG or antihuman IgM immunoglobulin in agar were purchased from Hyland Laboratories, Los Angeles, Calif. The lower limit of sensitivity of radial immunodiffusion for C1q, IgG and IgM plates was approximately 2 μg N/ml of C1q, 10 μg/ml protein of IgG and 5 μg/ml protein of IgM, respectively, although the standard curves for the immunoglobulins were non-linear at the lower concentrations.

Latex C1q test. This was carried out using the agglutination method of Ewald and Schubart

13

(22), employing fraction II-coated latex particles. The usual buffer was EDTA-glycine saline as described by these authors.

Acrylamide gel disc electrophoresis. This was carried out according to a modification of the method of Davis (23). Concentrations of 3.75% and 1.5% polyacrylamide were used for running gels and concentrating gels, respectively. Gel and electrode buffer contained 0.1% SDS. For analytic purposes, running gel measured 0.5 x 4.0 cm, and concentrating gel, 0.5 x 1.0 cm. For preparative purposes, 1.1 x 5.5 cm of running gel and 1.1 x 1.5 cm of concentrating gel were used. Usually, 0.1 or 0.05 ml of the sample, containing 0.75% SDS and 10% sucrose, was applied to the top of the smaller gel and 0.4 ml of sample was applied to the top of the larger gel. For studies of the subunits of C1q, gels containing 0.5 M urea and 0.1% SDS as described by Williamson *et al.* (24) were used at pH 7.2.

Rapid quantitative hemolytic assay for C1q. Using a Pasteur pipette, 1 drop of sample was mixed with an equal volume of sufficient Ca^{++} to neutralize EDTA, and then 1 drop containing an excess of purified C1r and C1s was added. After incubation for 15 min at 30°C to form macromolecular C1a, 1 drop of EAC4 (1×10^9 cells/ml) was added to the reaction mixtures and these mixtures were incubated at 30°C for 15 min to form SAC$\bar{1}$4. These cells were washed twice with DGVB^{++} to eliminate any unreacted C1r and C1s and resuspended in 0.5 ml of the same buffer, and then 1 drop of C2 (50 site-forming units (SFU)/cell) was added. After incubation at 30°C for 10 min, 1.5 ml of C-EDTA was added, and the reaction mixtures were incubated at 37°C for 30 min. The tubes were centrifuged, and the degree of hemolysis was graded from 0 (no detectable lysis) to 4+ (complete lysis).

Titration of C1q. The ability of several dilutions of C1q samples to form C$\bar{1}$ was determined by incubating C1q with constant amounts of C1r and C1s. The number of effective C1 molecules formed was determined by the method of Borsos and Rapp (19) after thoroughly washing the EAC$\bar{1}$4 cells with DGVB^{++} (RSC = 0.065) before C2 was added. Although we have used this assay to determine whether or not purified C1q is biologically active and have recorded specific activities using these conditions, final assessment of the specific activities of C1q will be reported at a later date. More complete knowledge of the number of subunits of C1q in a C1 molecule and the stability of its biologic activity is necessary.

N-determination. This was carried out with a modification of the Nesslerzation and Kjeldahl digestion method as described in (25). Three preparations of C1q were analyzed for nitrogen content.

Molecular weight estimation of C1q. Molecular weight was estimated according to a modification of the method of Dunker and Rueckert (26). Human serum albumin, human IgG and catalase were used as markers.

I. Purification of C1q

1. Pilot study: precipitation of C1q at various EGTA or EDTA concentrations. Three-milliliter portions of fresh serum were dialyzed against 250 ml of various concentrations of EGTA (RSC 0.020, 0.040, 0.060 and 0.076) at pH 7.5. Two-milliliter amounts of the same serum were dialyzed against 250 ml of EDTA (RSC 0.037 and 0.089) at pH 7.5, 0 to 4°C. After 19 hr, the resulting precipitates were collected by centrifugation at 10,000 × G for 20 min at 0 to 4°C, washed twice with the same buffer used for dialysis and dissolved with 0.3 M NaCl containing 0.01 M EDTA and 0.005 M phosphate buffer at pH 7.5. Two milliliters of the separated supernatants were dialyzed again for 17 hr using the same buffers and the precipitates were collected. All the separated supernatants and dissolved precipitates (after the first 19-hr dialysis period) were assayed for C1q, IgG and IgM using RID. The results are shown in Table I. The second dialysis period yielded slightly more C1q at RSC values of 0.060 and 0.076. C1q apparently is one of the least soluble serum proteins using these conditions. Essentially all the C1q was precipitated by EGTA or EDTA at a relative salt concentration lower than 0.04. Generally, precipitates made with EGTA buffers contain fewer contaminating serum proteins at similar RSC's. The analytic acryl-

TABLE I

Precipitation of C1q, IgG and IgM in EGTA at pH 7.5

	0.018 M; RSC, 0.020			0.034 M; RSC, 0.040			0.051 M; RSC, 0.060			0.065 M; RSC, 0.076		
	C1q	IgG	IgM	C1q	IgG	IgM	C1q	IgG	IgM	C1q	IgG	IgM
Total amount in original serum[a] μg N	61.8	4800	403.2	61.8	4800	403.2	61.8	4800	403.2	61.8	4800	403.2
Total amount precipitated[b] %	100.0	16.5	38.5	83.0	16.5	10.6	47.0	9.0	4.0	12.0	2.0	0
Amount recovered in precipitate[c] μg N	93.6[d]	46.1	15.4	52.7	19.4	9.1	11.1	15.0	<0.8	2.0	<1.6	<0.8

[a] After storage of the starting serum at 0°C for about 3 days.

[b] These figures represent the percentage of each protein precipitated from the starting serum. The amount in the supernatant after dialysis was subtracted from the starting serum value.

[c] The figures show the total amount contained in the precipitates recovered after dialysis for 19 hr, and after washing.

[d] The value is greater than the original serum, as in stored whole serum C1q is labile by radial immunodiffusion (28).

16

amide gel patterns of the redissolved precipitates are shown in Figure 1. Relatively less IgG and IgM was precipitated at the higher EDTA or EGTA concentrations. It was possible to choose optimal conditions for purification from this pilot study and longer dialysis times were indicated.

2. Purification of C1q for immunization. For purification of C1q to be used for antigenic stimulation the precipitate, obtained by dialysis of fresh whole human serum against 0.034 M EGTA (RSC = 0.04 at pH 7.5), for about 40 to 48 hr in the cold, was washed twice with the same EGTA solution. This precipitate was usually dissolved in one-tenth of the original serum volume with 0.3 M NaCl in 0.005 M phosphate buffer and 0.01 M EDTA (pH 7.5), and its optical density at 280 nm (OD$_{280}$) was approximately 2.0 (as measured in 0.1% SDS). On immunoelectrophoresis three to five precipitating lines against anti-whole human serum were found (Fig. 2).

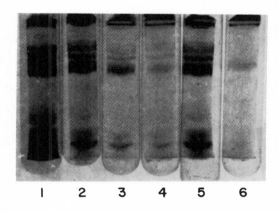

Figure 1. Acrylamide gel disc electrophoresis of human serum precipitates obtained by dialysis for 19 hr against various concentration of EGTA or EDTA, pH 7.5. Cathode is at the *top* (gel origin). Gel 1, 0.018 M EGTA (RSC = 0.020); gel 2, 0.034 M EGTA (RSC = 0.040); gel 3, 0.051 M EGTA (RSC = 0.060); gel 4, 0.065 M EGTA (RSC = 0.076); gel 5, 0.014 M EDTA (RSC = 0.037); and gel 6, 0.032 M EDTA (RSC = 0.089). C1q is the wide band migrating through approximately 1.4 cm of the length of the running gel (4 cm). It is the only band seen in gel 6.

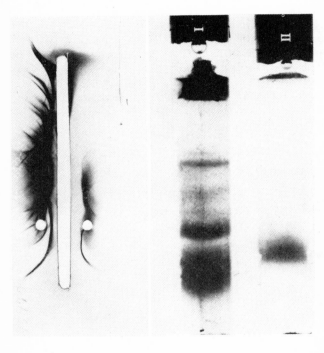

Figure 2. Purification of C1q for immunization. The *upper frame* shows immunoelectrophoresis of the single precipitated crude C1q used for further purification by acrylamide electrophoresis. *Upper well, whole human serum; lower well,* precipitate obtained by dialysis against 0.034 M EGTA, pH 7.5 RSC = 0.04, for 40 to 48 hr at 4°C; *trough,* horse anti-whole human serum. The anode is at the *right.* The *lower frame* shows the results of preparative acrylamide gel disc electrophoresis of the precipitate shown in the *upper frame.* Gel I, first electrophoretic run; gel II, second electrophoretic run. The applied sample was the gel segment from the first run which contained C1q.

Therefore, for further purification, two identical acrylamide gels were prepared and 0.4 ml of dissolved precipitate was applied to each. Electrophoresis was carried out with 65 V for the first 30 min and with 120 V for another 310 min using the preparative gels. After electrophoresis one of the gels was cut into 2-mm segments and kept in a humidity chamber until the position of C1q was located.

In order to locate C1q a longitudinal portion of the other gel from this run (gel I, Fig. 2) was fixed with 20% sulfosalicylic acid overnight, then fixed again with 20% trichloroacetic acid for 2 to 4 hr before staining. A second portion was cut into segments of 2 mm and eluted with 0.2 ml of 0.08 M NaCl in 0.1 M Tris-HCl buffer, pH 7.5, with continuous shaking at room temperature. After 60 min of elution, the latex agglutination activity of the eluate was assayed, and after 12 hr of elution, Ouchterlony double diffusion of each eluate against anti-whole human serum and anti-C1q (gift of Dr. H. J. Müller-Eberhard and Dr. R. J. Pickering) was carried out. As the latex agglutination activity after exposure to buffers containing SDS is relatively insensitive, the segments containing C1q were most efficiently located by examination of the stained gel segment (Fig. 2) and/or by Ouchterlony analysis.

The segment of the gel kept in a humidity chamber which corresponded to the C1q segment of gel I Figure 2 was placed on the top of a second acrylamide gel preparation after application of 0.1 ml of 0.75% SDS in 10% sucrose. After electrophoresis with the same conditions, one-eighth portion of this second run gel (gel II, Fig. 2) was cut longitudinally for staining, and the remaining portions were cut into 2-mm segments. Each segment was eluted by shaking with 0.3 ml of 0.08 M NaCl in 0.1 M Tris-HCl buffer (pH 7.5.) The gel segment containing C1q on this second run was identified by staining a quarter segment. The first and second runs are shown in Figure 2. C1q corresponded to the largest staining band on both the first and second gels. These segments also contained latex-agglutinating activity.

The eluates containing C1q after the second run were pulverized with their respective gel segments and mixed with equal volumes of Freund's complete adjuvant.

Each rabbit was immunized ·with approximately 100 μg of C1q (eluate from gel segments after two electrophoresis runs) in Freund's adjuvant. Injections were given directly into both popliteal nodes and subcutaneously or intradermally into the hip region. After 3 weeks, rabbits were bled and antibody content was estimated by Ouchterlony double diffusion against whole human serum. After 1 more week, each rabbit was boosted intradermally with 20 to 40 μg of C1q protein mixed with an equal volume of Freund's complete adjuvant. Approximately 3 weeks after the first immunization, rabbits began to produce strong precipitating anti-C1q antibodies.

II. Antibody to C1q

1. *Monospecificity of antibody.* As shown in Figure 3, by use of Ouchterlony double diffusion, the anti-C1q antiserum showed one precipitation line against whole human serum and against the purified C1q preparation. The antiserum did not exhibit any precipitation line against whole human serum or a purified C1q preparation inactivated at 56°C for 60 min.

As also shown in Figure 3, this antiserum shows one single precipitation arc in the slow γ-region on immunoelectrophoresis when run against purified C1q and one weak precipitation arc at the origin against whole human serum. The difference of mobility on the immunoelectrophoresis plate between purified C1q preparation and whole human serum may be due to interaction of C1q with IgG or IgM.

2. *Agglutination of EAC1q by anti-C1q.* One drop of whole human serum (17 μg N/ml of C1q) or purified C1q (19.5 μg N/ml of C1q) diluted serially in 0.01 M EDTA DGVB (RSC = 0.065) was mixed with 1 drop of EA in the same buffer (2 × 10^8 cells/ml in same buffer) in the wells of microtiter plates. After 20 min of incubation at 37°C, 1 drop of serially diluted antiserum (heat inactivated at 56°C for 60 min) and 1 drop of the same buffer were added. The plates were agitated for 5 min at room temperature and then held at 37°C for another 60 min. The degree of agglutination was graded from 0 (no visible agglutination) to 4 (strong agglutination).

As shown in Figure 4, this antiserum agglutinated EAC1q cells but did not agglutinate EA.

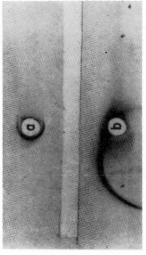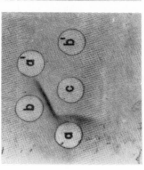

Figure 3. Monospecificity of rabbit anti-human C1q. *Left*, Ouchterlony double diffusion; *right*, immunoelectrophoresis (anode is to the *right*). *Well a*, whole human serum; *well b*, purified C1q; *well a'*, whole human serum treated at 56°C for 60 min; and *well b'*, purified C1q treated at 56°C for 60 min. *Well c and trough*, rabbit anti-human C1q.

21

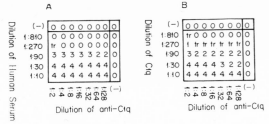

Figure 4. Agglutination of EAC1q by anti-C1q in EDTA-DGVB. The agglutination was carried out in microtiter plates. Rabbit anti-C1q was diluted as shown. *A*, EAC1q made with fresh human serum, diluted as shown. *B*, EAC1q made with purified C1q, diluted as shown. The degree of agglutination was graded from 0 (no detectable agglutination) to 4 (strong agglutination); tr, trace of agglutination.

III. *Isolation and purification of C1q using a combination of precipitation methods*

With increasing knowledge about the solubility of C1q, we were able to obtain highly purified C1q by three successive precipitation steps. The results of a typical purification run are outlined in Table II.

One hundred twenty-seven milliliters of fresh serum were dialyzed against 1000 ml of 0.026 M EGTA (RSC = 0.03, pH 7.5) for 4 hr at 4°C. The buffer was changed and dialysis was continued for another 11 hr. After dialysis for 15 hr the precipitate was separated, washed once with the same EGTA solution and dissolved with 32 ml of 0.75 M NaCl in 0.02 M acetate buffer containing 0.01 M EDTA (RSC = 0.80, pH 5.0). Insoluble aggregates were eliminated by centrifugation. The clear solution was dialyzed against 4000 ml of 0.06 M EDTA (RSC = 0.065, pH 5.0) for another 4 hr in the cold. The contents of the dialysis bag were centrifuged and the precipitate was separated. After this precipitate was washed, it was dissolved with 32 ml of 0.75 M NaCl in 0.005 M phosphate buffer containing 0.01 M EDTA (RSC = 0.80, pH 7.5) and was again centrifuged to eliminate insoluble aggregates. The clear solution was dialyzed against 4000 ml of 0.035 M EDTA (RSC = 0.069, pH 7.5) for 5 hr in the cold. After dialysis, the precipitate was separated

TABLE II

Summary of C1q purification (preparation 071670)

Procedures	Volume	OD$_{280}$ nm (%)	C1q μg N/ml (%)	IgG μg protein/ml (%)	IgM μg protein/ml (%)
Normal human serum[a]	126 ml	64.7 (100.0)	13.8 (100.0)	8600 (100)	1150 (100)
Supernatant of first dialysis	126	60.0 (92.7)	<2	NT[b]	NT
Precipitate of first dialysis	32	1.54 (0.604)	60.8 (>100.0)[c]	275 (8.12)	170 (3.75)
Supernatant of second dialysis	32	0.950 (0.373)	<2	NT	NT
Precipitate of second dialysis	32	0.529 (0.208)	51.2 (94.22)	<10 (<0.03)	9 (0.0099)
Supernatant of third dialysis	32	0.207 (0.0813)	<2	NT	NT
Precipitate of third dialysis	16	0.401 (0.0787)	74.0 (68.09)	<10 (<0.03)	<5 (<0.05)

[a] Starting normal human serum was kept at 0°C for about 2 days.
[b] NT, not tested.
[c] Recovery after the first precipitation is greater than 100% because of loss of antigenicity of the stored serum (28).

by centrifugation and was washed once with the same EDTA solution and then redissolved to 16 ml of 0.75 M NaCl in 0.02 M acetate buffer containing 0.01 M EDTA (RSC = 0.80, pH 7.5). A small portion was saved at each precipitation step to assay for C1q, IgG and IgM using RID.

As shown in Table II, the final yield of preparation 071670 was estimated to be 68%. This precipitation did not contain detectable IgG, IgM or IgA by RID. As shown in Figure 5, only one single precipitation arc in the slow γ-region against anti-whole human serum was seen on immunoelectrophoresis. Latex agglutination and hemolytic activity of C1q were found in the corresponding region of the agarose immunoelectrophoresis slide. This preparation showed only one major staining band on analytic acrylamide gel electrophoresis (Fig. 5). Generally the C1q obtained after two successive precipitations shows only one precipitation line against anti-whole human serum on immunoelectrophoresis and on Ouchterlony double diffusion. However, these preparations contain faint bands near the C1q band on analytic acrylamide gel electrophoresis, and these are negligible after the third precipitation.

1. Hemolytic activity of C1q. To 0.2 ml of serial dilutions of purified C1q in DGVB^{++} (RSC = 0.065, pH = 7.4) 0.3 ml of a reagent containing constant amounts of C1r (1.95×10^{10} effective molecules/ml) and C1s ($0.4 \mu g/ml$) was added.

After incubation at 30°C for 45 min, 0.25-ml portions were transferred into the test tubes containing equal volumes of EAC4 (1.5×10^8 cells/ml in the same buffer). These reaction mixtures were incubated at 30°C for 45 min and the cells were washed three times with the same buffer. The test tubes were changed once during this washing step to wash away residual free C1s and C1r. The washed cells were resuspended to 0.75 ml with diluted C2 (to give 62 SFU/cell) and were incubated at 30°C for 10 min. After the addition of 3.0 ml of 1/50 C-EDTA, the samples were then incubated at 37°C for 90 min. The percentage of cells hemolyzed was determined spectrophotometrically and the number of C1 molecules calculated according to Borsos and Rapp (19). As shown in Figure 6, the purified C1q, stored at

24

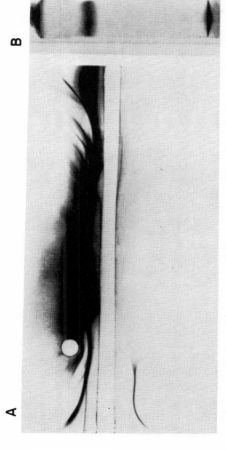

Figure 5. Purity of C1q (preparation 071670). *A,* immunoelectrophoresis (anode is to the *right*). *Upper well,* normal whole human serum; *lower well,* purified C1q; and *trough,* horse anti-whole human serum. *B,* Acrylamide gel disc electrophoresis, pH 8.6. Applied sample was 0.1 ml of C1q (37 μg N/ml) obtained by three precipitation steps.

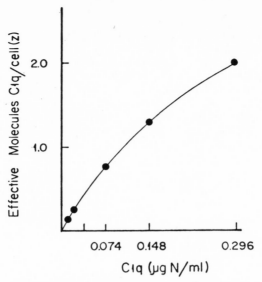

Effective Molecules C1q/cell (z)

2.0

1.0

0.074   0.148   0.296

C1q (μg N/ml)

Figure 6. Hemolytic activity of C1q (preparation 071670). The hemolytic activity of C1q purified by precipitation was tested by incubating
various concentrations of C1q and a reagent containing C1r and C1s (see text) in the presence of
Ca^{++} at 30°C for 45 min, followed by addition of
EAC4. After the incubation at 30°C for 45 min
and washing, the resulting SAC$\overline{1}$4 were assayed
according to Borsos and Rapp (19).

0°C for about 2 weeks, showed that 0.069 μg N of
C1q gave 1.5×10^8 effective molecules of C$\overline{1}$. The
relatively low specific activity may reflect less
than optimal titration conditions and the lability
of C1q. The lability of C1q (antigenically and
functionally) will have to be controlled before
higher specific activities are obtained.

This purified C1q preparation did not contain
any detectable C1r and C1s by specific assays as
described (16, 17).

2. Latex agglutination activity of purified C1q.
Twofold serial dilutions of 0.25 ml of purified C1q
(74 μg N/ml as C1q) were made in 0.01 M EDTA-
glycine saline and in VBS^{++}. Another series of
dilutions was made in the same buffers containing
3% albumin. An equal volume of fraction II-
coated latex particles was added to each tube and
mixed. After incubation at room temperature for

2 hr, the degree of agglutination was graded from 0 (no agglutination detected) to 4 + (strong agglutination detected). Alternatively, the reactions may be held in the cold overnight before agglutination patterns are read.

The latex agglutination titer of purified C1q was 1:80 and the amount of C1q nitrogen at the end point was 0.93 μg N/ml, using 0.01 M EDTA-glycine saline or VBS++. Using 0.01 M EDTA-glycine saline or VBS++ containing 3% albumin, the agglutination titers of purified C1q increased to 1:320 (0.23 μg N/ml). This change in functional activity suggests that purified C1q may change its conformation in high salt, in high concentrations of chelating chemicals and on aging. These changes may be partially reversible. The enhancing effect of albumin may be caused by decreased nonspecific protein surface interactions

IV. Estimation of molecular weight of C1q and subunits of C1q

Purified C1q elutes in the void volume on Sephadex G-200 and its molecular weight has been estimated to be 400,000 (8). Our studies of molecular weight used the method of relative mobility in acrylamide electrophoresis (26).

Purified C1q, 0.05 ml, was applied to 4% acrylamide gels containing 0.1% SDS. Human serum albumin, human γ globulin and catalase were used as markers with known molecular weights of 69,000, 160,000 and 240,000, respectively. After the electrophoretic run the gels were stained and the relative mobilities were calculated using the buffer interface as a reference point.

As shown in Table III, the average molecular weight of purified C1q on six runs was 387,600 ± 10,790.

As a result of experiments designed to study the mobility of C1q in buffers of varying composition and after reduction and alkylation, lower molecular weight subunits were discovered. As shown in Figure 7, using 0.5 M urea at pH 7.2 and using L and H chains from IgM and IgG as markers, subunits with an estimated molecular weight of approximately 60,000 and 40,000 were noted. Also after reduction with 0.1 M dithiothreitol, followed by iodoacetamide (0.15 M), two subunits with an approximate molecular weight of 30,000

27

TABLE III
Estimation of molecular weight of C1q[a]

Gel No.	Relative Mobility				Calculated m.w. of C1q
	Albumin	γG	Catalase	C1q	
Gel I	0.930	0.853	0.605	0.318	385,000
Gel II	0.930	0.853	0.612	0.318	395,000
Gel III	0.934	0.868	0.625	0.338	401,000
Gel IV	0.933	0.859	0.622	0.333	395,000
	Albumin monomer	Albumin dimer	Albumin trimer	C1q	
Gel V	0.922	0.690	0.512	0.310	375,000
Gel VI	0.944	0.710	0.521	0.340	375,000

[a] The relative mobility of the protein markers and C1q were measured in relation to the buffer front. A 4% gel, pH 8.6, 0.1% SDS was used. The molecular weights of the markers are given in the text.

and 20,000 were noted (Fig. 7). These experiments will be reported in more detail later; however, we feel that C1q may have a non-covalent subunit structure although some intact C1q is still present in 0.5 M urea (Fig. 7). The electron microphotographs of C1q by Svehag and Bloth (27) suggest a similar subunit by direct dimensional measurement. As C1q is an important link between immunoglobulins and the biologic activities of the complement system, further biochemical study is in progress.

DISCUSSION

The purification of C1q has been difficult because of its minimal solubility at low ionic strength and the lability of its biologic activity (2) and antigenicity (28). Consequently, large amounts are lost with usual column chromatographic and zone electrophoretic methods. The purification scheme described herein is simple and takes advantage of this insolubility to increase yields. Highly purified C1q can be obtained by repeated precipitation in the presence of chelating agents to eliminate C1r and C1s. The final yield is approximately 40 to 60%. Alternatively, C1q can be highly purified for antigenic stimulation after a

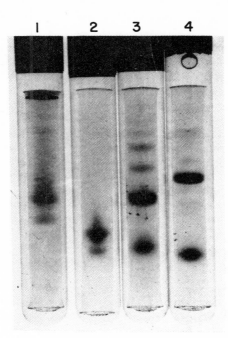

Figure 7. Acrylamide electrophoresis of purified Clq in 0.5 M urea, 0.1% SDS, pH 7.2. Gel 1, Clq (071670) (for comparison without urea see Figure 5*B*); gel 2, Clq (071670), reduced and alkylated; gel 3, human IgG, reduced and alkylated; gel 4, human IgM, H and L chains separated by sulfitolysis.

single precipitation by using two identical acrylamide gel steps in a SDS buffer system. Monospecific antisera can be obtained by immunizing with the acrylamide gel segments containing Clq. The purified Clq that is obtained by precipitation has latex-agglutinating activity and hemolytic activity when mixed with Clr and Cls in the presence of Ca^{++}. These biologic activities, as well as the antigenicity of Clq, are labile on storage. The hemolytic titration of this preparation was based on its ability to form Cl molecules when added to optimal amounts of Clr and Cls (Fig. 6). Optimal conditions for maximal hemolytic activity are being studied.

This preparation will be useful in future investigations of Clq binding to antigen-antibody complexes, and it should be useful for detection of other proteins and substances in human serum and human disease states that react with C1q.

C1q is known to react with many other polyanionic substances in what is presumed to be a nonspecific fashion (14). These substances may be "anti-complementary" and whether or not the C system is activated in a biologically significant manner requires further study.

We are currently investigating the chemical structure of C1q with this preparation. Müller-Eberhard (8) has reported that C1q has an unusual amino acid composition and a high carbohydrate content. He has also suggested small subunits after reduction and alkylation. Our finding of small subunits (approximate molecular weight 40,000 to 60,000) after 0.5 M urea suggests an important non-covalent structure. Studies are in progress to describe in more detail the chemical structure of C1q.

REFERENCES

1. Lepow, I. H., Naff, G. B., Todd, W. D., Pensky, J. and Hinz, C. F., J. Exp. Med., *117:* 983, 1963.
2. Müller-Eberhard, H. J. and Kunkel, H. G., Proc. Soc. Exp. Biol. Med., *106:* 291, 1960.
3. Weigle, W. O. and Maurer, P. H., J. Immun., *79:* 211, 1957.
4. Paul, W. E. and Benacerraf, B., J. Immun., *95:* 1067, 1966.
5. Thunold, S., Abeyounis, C. J. and Milgrom, F., J. Immun., *104:* 685, 1970.
6. Ratnoff, O. D. and Naff, G. B., J. Exp. Med., *125:* 337, 1967.
7. Naff, G. B. and Ratnoff, O. D., J. Exp. Med., *128:* 571, 1968.
8. Müller-Eberhard, H. J., Advances Immun., *8:* 1–80, 1968.
9. Linscott, W. D. and Hansen, S. S., J. Immun., *103:* 423, 1969.
10. Borsos, T. and Rapp, H. J., Science, *150:* 505, 1965.
11. Linscott, W. D., J. Immun., *102:* 1322, 1969.
12. Hyslop, N. E. Jr., Dourmashkin, R. R., Green, N. M. and Porter, R. R., J. Exp. Med., *131:* 783, 1970.
13. Müller-Eberhard, H. J., Ann. Rev. Biochem., *38:* 389, 1969.
14. Agnello, V., Carr, R. I., Koffler, K. and Kunkel, H. G., Fed. Proc., *28:* 696, 1969.

15. Nelson, R. A., Jr., Jensen, J., Gigli, I. and Tamura, N., Immunochemistry, *3:* 111, 1966.
16. deBracco, M. and Stroud, R. M., J. Clin. Invest., In press.
17. Nagaki, K. and Stroud, R. M., J. Immun., *102:* 421, 1969.
18. Mayer, M. M., in *Kabat and Mayer's Experimental Immunochemistry*, 2nd Ed., Charles C Thomas, Springfield, Ill., 1961.
19. Borsos, T. and Rapp, H. J., J. Immun., *91:* 851, 1963.
20. Scheidegger, J. J., Int. Arch. Allerg., *7:* 103, 1955.
21. Mancini, G., Carbonara, A. O. and Heremans, J. F., Immunochemistry, *2:* 235, 1965.
22. Ewald, R. W. and Schubart, A. F., J. Immun., *97:* 100, 1966.
23. Davis, B. J., Ann. N. Y. Acad. Sci., *121:* 304, 1964.
24. Williamson, A. R. and Askonas, B. A., Biochem. J., *107:* 823, 1968.
25. Chase, M. W. and Williams, C. A., in *Methods in Immunology and Immunochemistry*, Vol. II, Academic Press, New York and London, 1968.
26. Dunker, A. K. and Rueckert, R. R., J. Biol. Chem., *244:* 5074, 1969.
27. Svehag, S. and Bloth, B., Acta Path. Microbiol. Scand. Section B, *78:* 260, 1970.
28. Hanauer, L. B. and Christian, C. L., Amer. J. Med., *42:* 882, 1967.

PURIFICATION OF THE HUMAN COMPLEMENT PROTEIN Clq BY AFFINITY CHROMATOGRAPHY

Carlos R. Sledge and David H. Bing

A subunit of the first component of human complement Clq, was puri-fied by the technique of affinity chromatography. The chromatographic resin was cyanogen bromide-activated Sepharose covalently linked to hu-man IgG. For the removal of traces of IgM it was necessary to subject further the Clq obtained from the chromatographic step to ultracentrifu-gation in sucrose gradients. The highly purified Clq was characterized im-munochemically and according to its electrophoretic mobility in poly-acrylamide gel. The purified material was capable of combining with Clr and Cls to reconstitute fully active macromolecular Cl.

The first component of human complement is composed of three distinct proteins, Clq, Clr, and Cls,[2] which associate physically in the

[1] This work was supported by Public Health Ser-vice Pre-doctoral Training Grant GM 01911-04 and Public Health Service Grant 1-ROI-AM-13679-03 from the National Institutes of Health. This is Jour-nal Article No. 5935 from the Michigan Agricultural Experiment Station.

[2] The terminology used for the complement pro-teins is that suggested in the Bull. Wld. Hlth. Org. "Nomenclature of Complement," Immunochemistry, 7: 137, 1970. Complement components are designated numerically C1, C2, C3, C4, C5, C6, C7, C8 and C9; the subunits of C1 are designated Clq, Clr and Cls; activated components are designated by placing a rule over the numeral which refers to the component or subunit. Cellular intermediates carrying comple-ment components are designated EAC, followed by the numeral designating the components carried, e.g., EACĪ,4. CEDTA is serum diluted in ethylenedi-amine tetraacetic acid. TBS is triethanolamine-buf-fered saline and TB-sucrose is triethanolamine-buf-fered sucrose.

presence of calcium ion to form fully active macromolecular $\overline{C1}$. C1q binds to the antibody molecule of an antigen-antibody complex, and initiates the sequence of events involved in complement-mediated immunecytolysis (1, 2). The nature of the interaction of C1q with immunoglobulins apparently involves the following parameters: 1) only IgG and IgM will combine with $\overline{C1}$q (3, 4), 2) the binding site for C1q is in the Fc region (2), and 3) the C1q-immunoglobulin complex can be dissociated by low pH-high ionic strength salt solutions and diaminoalkyl compounds (5, 6).

The preceding information suggested that an affinity chromatographic procedure for C1q could be developed based on adsorption to IgG covalently linked to a resin and elution with a suitable diaminoalkyl compound. This report presents evidence that this can be accomplished and that the technique is a rapid, reproducible method for obtaining milligram quantities of highly purified C1q from a few hundred milliliters of whole serum.

MATERIALS AND METHODS

Chemicals and reagents. All chemicals and solvents were reagent grade. Triple distilled water was used for all buffers. 1,4-Diaminobutane was obtained as the free base from Aldrich Chemical Co. (Milwaukee, Wis.). Hemolysin was obtained from Behring Diagnostics (Woodbury, N. Y.). Sheep blood, from a single male sheep, was collected into Alsever's solution. Guinea pig blood and pooled human serum were donated by the Michigan State Public Health Laboratories (Lansing, Mich.).

Chemical procedures. The procedure of Bing (7) was used to link covalently human IgG to 40 ml of settled Sepharose. By assuming an extinction of 1.5 for a 1 mg/ml solution of IgG (8), it was determined that 370.6 mg of protein had been bound to the resin. The resin was then washed exhaustively with 0.075 ionic strength Tris-HCl-0.01 M EDTA, pH 8.1, and stored at 4°C with 0.005 M sodium azide as a preservative. Protein concentrations were also determined by the method of Lowry *et al.* (9).

Crystalline bovine serum albumin was used to construct a standard curve.

Protein preparations. Human IgG was isolated from pooled human serum by chromatography on DEAE-cellulose (10), and by precipitation with $(NH_4)_2SO_4$ at 40% saturation. It contained only IgG immunoglobulin according to immunoelectrophoretic analysis with a rabbit anti-whole human serum antiserum. The low ionic strength acid precipitate (euglobulin fraction) of serum was prepared by precipitation of human serum with 0.02 ionic strength acetate buffer (pH 5.5) to yield a final serum ionic strength of 0.03 and a pH of 6.4 (1). The precipitate was redissolved in 0.3 M NaCl to one-tenth the original serum volume and dialyzed for 18 hr against two 1-liter changes of 0.1 ionic strength Tris-HCl-0.01 M EDTA, pH 8.1. The protein was centrifuged 30 min at 10,000 rpm (12,100 $\times$ G) before application to the column.

A reagent deficient in C1q (RC1q), but containing C1r and C1s, was prepared by incubation of 5 ml of euglobulin precipitate with 50 ml of IgG Sepharose resin for 15 hr at 4°C. The resin was then poured into a column and eluted with 0.075 ionic strength Tris-HCl-0.01 M EDTA. The eluate was judged to be depleted of C1q by its inability to form $EAC\overline{1},4$ cells (11). Functionally pure C1q, C1r, and C1s were generously provided by Dr. I. H. Lepow, Department of Pathology, University of Connecticut Health Center, Farmington, Conn.

Assays. $EAC\overline{1},4$ cells were prepared by the method of Mayer (12), except 0.15 ionic strength triethanolamine-buffered saline (TBS), pH 7.4 (13), was substituted for Veronal-buffered saline. EAC4 cells were obtained by incubation overnight at 4°C in pH 7.4, 0.15 ionic strength, TBS containing 0.01 M EDTA (12). The hemolytic activity of C1q was determined by its ability to form macromolecular C1 when varying concentrations of C1q were added to a constant amount of the C1r and C1s or the RC1q reagent in the presence of 0.02 M $CaCl_2$ according to the following modifications and procedures: C1q was added to a mixture of C1r and C1s or RC1q diluted in 0.065 ionic strength triethanolamine-buffered sucrose (TB sucrose), pH 7.4 (13), in the presence of 0.02 M $CaCl_2$ and incubated at 37°C for 10 min. The dilution of C1q and RC1q was determined by cross-titration of each reagent with functionally pure C1q, C1r, and C1s. Then 0.1 ml of each dilution was added to 0.1 ml of EAC4 (1.5×10^8 cells/ml) in 0.065 ionic strength TB-sucrose, and incubation was continued for 10 min at 37°C. The resulting $EAC\overline{1},4$ intermediate was centrifuged and washed three times with warm 0.065 ionic strength TB-sucrose. The cells were then transferred to a new tube and 0.1 ml of C2 was added to provide 50 to 100 effective molecules per cell (13). After incubation at 30°C for 10 min with shaking, 1.2 ml of CEDTA (a 1:25 dilution of serum) was added and incubation was continued at 37°C for 60 min. The degree of lysis was measured at 412 nm, and effective molecules were calculated as previously described (11). Guinea pig C2 and guinea pig serum was used in all cases for measurement of C1 activity. C1q activity was also detected by the slide agglutination test of Ewald and Schubert (14) with fraction II γ globulin-coated latex particles.

Affinity chromatography using IgG-Sepharose. A 2.5- x 9.0-cm column of IgG-Sepharose was poured and equilibrated at 4°C with 0.075 ionic strength Tris-HCl + 0.01 M EDTA, pH 8.1. Six milliliters of euglobulin fraction in 0.1 ionic strength Tris-HCl + 0.01 M EDTA, pH 8.1, were applied to the column and 4-ml fractions collected. The column was washed with equilibration buffer until the absorbancy at 280 nm of the effluent was less than 0.05. The column was then eluted with 0.4 M NaCl + 0.01 M EDTA until the absorbancy of the effluent at 280 nm was less than 0.05. Finally the column was eluted with 0.2 M 1,4-diaminobutane. Tubes containing protein were pooled and dialyzed against 0.15 ionic strength Tris-HCl + 0.01 M EDTA, pH 8.1.

Ultracentrifugation. A Beckman model L2-65B ultracentrifuge and an SW27 rotor were used for the sucrose gradient ultracentrifugation. The sample was layered on a linear 10 to 40% (w/v) sucrose gradient buffered with 0.5

ionic strength acetate, pH 5.0. Centrifugation was conducted for 15 hr at 27,000 rpm, 4°C. Fifty-drop fractions were collected.

Moving boundary sedimentation velocity experiments were carried out in the Spinco model E analytical ultracentrifuge at 3 to 5°C and a rotor speed of 56,000 rpm with an AN-D 2350 rotor. Pool q preparations were analyzed at a concentration of 5 mg/ml in both 0.15 ionic strength Tris-HCl, pH 8.1, and 0.5 ionic strength acetate, pH 5.0 buffers. Apparent sedimentation coefficients were corrected to 20°C.

Immunodiffusion analysis. Ouchterlony double diffusion was carried out in 0.5% agarose in 0.15 M NaCl containing 0.01 M EDTA and 0.1% sodium azide. Immunoelectrophoresis was conducted in 1% agarose (Nutritional Biochemical Corporation, Cleveland, Ohio) in 0.025 ionic strength Veronal buffer, pH 8.3, containing 0.01 M EDTA at 3 mA/slide for 40 min at 4°C (7). The pool q preparation was made 10 mg/ml and sucrose gradient purified C1q was made 5 mg/ml for analysis by immunodiffusion and immunoelectrophoresis.

Acrylamide gel analysis. Acrylamide gel electrophoresis was conducted in 5% gels at pH 8.3 at 2 mA/gel according to the procedure of Gabriel (15). The gel was fixed in 10% trichloroacetic acid and scanned at 280 nm with a Gilford gel scanner (Gilford Instruments, Oberlin, Ohio) at a slit width of 0.05 mm. One hundred fifty to 200 μg of protein were applied to the gel.

Antisera. Rabbit antisera against the euglobulin fraction and human serum were prepared as previously described (7).

RESULTS

Chromatography on IgG-Sepharose. The elution profile of the euglobulin fractions chromatographed on the IgG-Sepharose column is illustrated in Figure 1. The protein which had no binding affinity for the resin comprised pool A. Pool U represented nonspecifically bound protein eluted with 0.4 M NaCl + 0.01 M EDTA. The C1q was eluted in pool q with 0.2 M 1,4-diaminobutane. Table I summarizes the results of a typical experiment. The majority of the protein applied to the resin was not adsorbed and pool A represented 85.6% of the applied material. Pool q contained 2.7% of the protein in the euglobulin fraction. The ability of the various column fractions to agglutinate γ globulin-coated latex particles was determined. Pool A yielded a weakly positive reaction; pool U was negative; and pool q strongly agglutinated the latex particles. The pool q prepa-

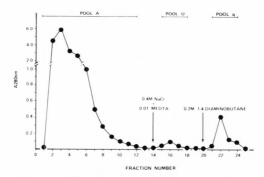

Figure 1. Chromatography of the euglobulin fraction of serum on IgG-Sepharose. The arrows indicate the points of addition of 0.4 M NaCl + 0.01 M EDTA and 0.2 M 1,4-diaminobutane.

TABLE I

Purification of C1q on IgG-Sepharose[a]

| Fraction | Volume | Protein | | Latex Agglutination |
		mg/ml	Total	
	ml			
Serum	60.0			+
Euglobulin	6.0	15.20	91.2	+
Pool A	65.0	1.20	78.0	±
Pool U	15.0	0.10	1.5	−
Pool q	20.0	0.12	2.4	+

[a] Protein concentration was determined by the method of Lowry *et al.* (9) as outlined in *Materials and Methods.*

rations did not contain any detectable C1s and C1r when tested by esterolytic assays with synthetic substrates (16, 17).

Ultracentrifugation. In the model E analyti-

37

cal ultracentrifuge at an ionic strength of 0.15 and a final speed of 56,060 rpm pool q contained a rapidly sedimenting peak with an s_{20} value greater than 30, and a well-defined peak with an s_{20} value of 10.2. When the same material was centrifuged under the same conditions in 0.5 ionic strength buffer, none of the $30S_{20}$ material was observed; rather two peaks of $10.2S_{20}$ and $17.8S_{20}$ appeared (data not shown).

It was decided to fractionate further pool q on a sucrose gradient to obtain the $10.2S_{20}$ protein free of the $17.8S_{20}$ material. Pool q preparations obtained from 30 ml of euglobulin were concentrated to 11 mg/ml and applied to a 10 to 40% sucrose gradient. Figure 2 is a profile of the gradient. Two species of protein are clearly evident sedimenting in the 19S and 10S region

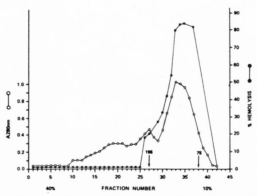

Figure 2. Ten to 40% sucrose gradient ultracentrifugation of pool q. O——O, A_{280} nm; ●——●, hemolytic activity.

of the gradient. The C1q activity, in terms of its ability to combine with the RC1q to form $\overline{C1}$ and lyse EAC4, was found to be associated with the protein in the 10S region. Fractions 30 to 38 were pooled and analyzed along with pool q according to their behavior in immunoelectrophoresis, immunodiffusion, and polyacrylamide electrophoresis. This preparation of C1q̄ represented 1.6% of the total protein originally in the euglobulin fractions applied to the IgG-Sepharose resin. The protein in the 19S region was determined to be IgM by immunodiffusion analysis with a rabbit antiserum to a human IgM.

Hemolytic activity of the isolated C1q. Various dilutions of sucrose gradient-purified C1q were incubated with a constant amount of C1r and C1s or the RC1q reagent (see *Materials and Methods*) in the presence of 0.02 M $CaCl_2$. The ability of these mixtures to lyse EAC4 upon the addition of the remaining complement components was determined and expressed as the number of effective C1 molecules/μg protein (Table II). According to both assays, lysis was

TABLE II
The ability of purified C1q to form $\overline{C1}$[a]

Reagent	μg C1q	Z	Effective Molecules/ μg Protein
C1r + C1s	0.087	0.465	1.04×10^{12}
	0.043	0.192	
RC1q	0.13	0.342	0.6×10^{12}
	0.050	0.186	

[a] Protein concentrations, Z, and effective molecules/μg protein were determined as outlined in *Materials and Methods*.

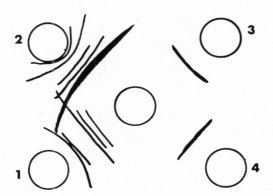

Figure 3. Immunodiffusion analysis. *Center well,* anti-whole human serum; *1,* human serum; *2,* euglobulin, 20 mg/ml; *3,* pool q, 1.5 mg/ml; *4,* purified C1q, 1.5 mg/ml.

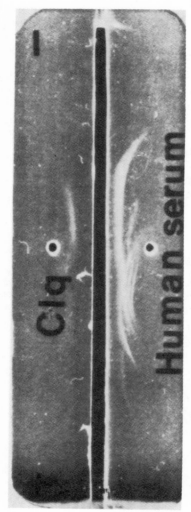

Figure 4. Immunoelectrophoresis of C1q and human serum. *Upper well,* C1q 1.5 mg/ml; *lower well,* human serum 5 μl; *trough,* rabbit anti-euglobulin fraction.

still detectable at a C1q concentration of less than 0.2 µg/ml, and the effective molecules per microgram of protein were comparable in both assays. The activity was expressed as effective molecules per microgram to provide comparison with previously published reports on C1q (18).

Immunodiffusion. In gel diffusion analysis both pool q and C1q, purified further by ultracentrifugation in sucrose gradients, yielded single precipitin arcs upon reaction with a rabbit anti-human serum antiserum. In these experiments, pool q and C1q obtained from the preparative ultracentrifugation were analyzed at a concentration of 1.5 mg/ml (Fig. 3). The bands were visible at 18 hr but it was necessary to continue diffusion for 3 days refilling the wells each day to make the C1q precipitin line dense enough for photographic reproduction. The same preparation of C1q was also analyzed by immunoelectrophoresis with rabbit antiserum to the euglobulin fraction (Fig. 4). Only a single precipitin band in the γ region was detected even after 3 days of incubation at room temperature. Pool q reacted with a rabbit anti-human IgM antiserum in immunodiffusion analysis, but the gradient-purified C1q did not. Neither reacted with rabbit anti-human IgG antiserum.

The purified C1q and pool q were also analyzed according to electrophoretic mobility in a variety of polyacrylamide electrophoretic systems. In 5% acrylamide gels at pH 8.3 (Fig. 5), the gradient-purified C1q contained two

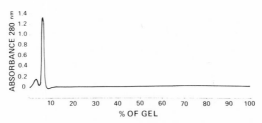

Figure 5. Scan of C1q in 5% polyacrylamide electrophoresis at pH 8.3. See *Materials and Methods* for experimental details.

41

bands. The more anodically migrating band represented 94.7% of the protein detectable in the gel. Because no IgM nor IgG could be detected in gradient-purified C1q and only one component could be detected immunochemically, it was postulated that a) the minor band detectable in 5% polyacrylamides at pH 8.3 was an aggregate and/or break down product of C1q resulting from the ammonium persulfate, the catalyst used in these systems, and b) the material in pool q which would not enter the running gels was IgM and/or IgM-C1q complexes detected in the sucrose gradient ultracentrifugation step.

DISCUSSION

Affinity chromatography offers a simple, reproducible technique for the purification of highly active, highly purified, C1q. The C1q obtained directly from the affinity chromatographic column was estimated to contain 92 to 95% C1q. Furthermore, this material combined with C1r and C1s or an RC1q reagent to form functional $C\overline{1}$ as detected with EAC4, C2, and CEDTA. In a similar assay with C1q purified by precipitation from serum, Yonemasu and Stroud (18) found that C1q only contained 1.5 $\times$ 10^8 effective molecules/μg N of protein. It was of some interest to compare our preparation with this previously published procedure. Even taking into account the differences in methods of protein determination, the C1q purified by affinity chromatography is considerably more active since it contained 1 to 0.6 $\times$ 10^{12} effective molecules/μg protein (Table II).

If the molecular weight of C1q is taken as 4×10^5 daltons then 1.2×10^{12} effective molecules equal about 1 μg of C1q if the efficiency of lysis is 100%. The present data indicate there are 1.04 $\times$ 10^{12} effective C1q molecules/μg and thus the overall efficiency of the affinity chromatographically purified C1q is approaching the overall efficiency of C1 which is 90 to 100% in the hemolytic assay (19). This further confirms the biochemical purity of the preparation. With this procedure 3 to 4 mg of highly purified C1q can be obtained from 100 ml of serum in about 2 days. This means the overall yield of C1q is

42

about 25%, if the C1q concentration in serum is taken at 0.15 μg/ml. The major loss is apparently in the affinity chromatographic step, in which there is an equilibrium situation between the IgG-Sepharose, the C1q, and probably the IgM present in the euglobulin fraction.

Fractionation of the pool q in a 10 to 40% sucrose gradient resulted in the separation of the contaminating IgM from the pool q. It was observed that if gradient ultracentrifugation was conducted at an ionic strength of 0.15, the majority of the protein sedimented to the bottom of the gradient (Sledge, unpublished results). However, if the ionic strength was raised to 0.5, then the 10.2S and 17.8S sedimenting components detected in the analytical ultracentrifuge were apparently separated in the 19S and 10S region of the sucrose gradient (Fig. 3), and the resulting C1q was free of any other identifiable serum proteins.

Acknowledgments. The authors gratefully acknowledge Dr. Kristine Knudson, Ms. Sandra Spurlock and Ms. Janice Mernitz for informative discussions, and Dr. Richard Patrick for his critical review of the manuscript.

REFERENCES

1. Lepow, I. H., Naff, G. W., Todd, E. W., Pensky, J., and Hinz, C. F., J. Exp. Med., *117:* 983, 1963.
2. Loos, M., Borsos, T., and Rapp, H. J., J. Immunol., *108:* 683, 1972.
3. Augener, W., Grey, H. M., Cooper, N. R., and Müller-Eberhard, H. J., Immunochemistry, *8:* 1011, 1971.
4. Morse, J. H. and Christian, C. L., J. Exp. Med., *119:* 195, 1963.
5. Müller-Eberhard, H. J., in *Advances in Immunology*, edited by F. J. Dixon, Jr., and H. G. Kunkel, Vol. 8, p. 2, Academic Press, New York, 1968.
6. Wirtz, G. H., Immunochemistry, *2:* 95, 1965.
7. Bing, D. H., J. Immunol., *107:* 1243, 1971.
8. McClure, W. O. and Edelman, G. M., Biochemistry, *5:* 1908, 1966.
9. Lowry, O. H., Rosebrough, N. J., Farr, A. L., and

Randall, R. J., J. Biol. Chem., *193:* 265, 1951.

10. Fahey, J. L., in *Methods in Immunology and Immunochemistry*, edited by C. A. Williams and M. W. Chase, Vol. 1, p. 322, Academic Press, New York, 1967.

11. Rapp, H. J. and Borsos, T., *Molecular Basis of Complement Action*, p. 90, Appleton-Century-Crofts, New York, 1970.

12. Kabat, E. A. and Mayer, M. M., in *Kabat and Mayer's Experimental Immunochemistry*, Chapter 4, Charles C Thomas, Springfield, Ill., 1961.

13. Bing, D. H., Mernitz, J. L., and Spurlock, S. E., Biochemistry, *11:* 4263, 1972.

14. Ewald, R. W. and Schubert, A. F., J. Immunol., *97:* 100, 1966.

15. Gabriel, O., in *Methods in Enzymology*, Edited by W. B. Jakoby, Vol. XXII, p. 565, Academic Press, New York, 1971.

16. Bing, D. H., Biochemistry, *8:* 4503, 1969.

17. Naff, G. B. and Ratnoff, O. D., J. Exp. Med., *128:* 571, 1969.

18. Yonemasu, K. and Stroud, R. M., J. Immunol., *106:* 304, 1971.

19. Colten, H. R., Borsos, T., and Rapp, H. J., Science, *158:* 1590, 1967.

44

PURIFICATION OF THE HUMAN COMPLEMENT PROTEIN C1s̄ BY AFFINITY CHROMATOGRAPHY*

DAVID H. BING

Abstract — Highly purified preparations of C1s̄, the esterase enzyme which is part of the macromolecular complex comprising C1, the first component of complement, can be obtained using the technique of affinity chromatography. The resin used was Sepharose coupled to meta-aminobenzamidine with cyanogen bromide. About 25 mg of C1s̄ is obtained from 200 ml of human serum. The enzyme obtained by this procedure has been characterized using immunochemical and enzymatic techniques. The protein reacts with anti-C1s̄ antiserum, causes formation of E* from EAC4, and is inhibitable by C1 inactivator, the naturally occurring serum inhibitor.

INTRODUCTION

Preparations of highly purified complement proteins can be obtained by employing ion exchange, adsorption, or gel filtration chromatographic procedures in combination with zonal centrifugational and preparative electrophoretic techniques (Müller–Eberhard, 1968; Shin and Mayer, 1968). With these techniques the yields of the various complement proteins range from 6 per cent for C3† to 0·5 per cent for C8 (Müller–Eberhard, 1968; Manni and Müller–Eberhard, 1969). For more detailed studies on the structure of the complement proteins it would be desirable to develop methods for obtaining in high yield homogeneous preparations of the complement proteins. For this reason, we decided to investigate the possibility of applying a new technique, termed affinity chromatography (Cuacatrecasas, 1968) to the purification of one well defined complement protein C1s̄.

The principle of affinity chromatography is similar to that underlying the use of immuno-adsorbents; the protein reacts specifically via its active site with a ligand, usually an inhibitor, covalently bound to a solid matrix. The specific nature of the active site of the protein enhances the reaction with resin. Elution of the protein from the resin is effected by adding free inhibitor or weak acid.

*Article No. 5211 from the Michigan Agricultural Experiment Station; supported by a grant from the National Institutes of Health, 1-ROI-AM-13679-02-ALY.

†The terminology used for the complement proteins is that suggested in the *Bull. Wld Hlth Org.* **39**, 935 (1968): C1s̄ is the enzymatically active form of C1s, the third subunit of the first component, C1, of human complement. The other subunits of C1 are C1q and C1r. C2, C3 and C4 are the second, third and fourth components of complement respectively. EA are sheep erythrocytes treated with antisheep erythrocyte antiserum. E* represents the complement-lysed EA. C1 inactivator is the naturally occurring serum inhibitor of C1s̄.

The unique aspect of affinity chromatography is that the resins have an extremely high capacity and there is usually a large yield of purified material (Cuacatrecasas, 1970). The method has wide applicability as it has recently been successfully employed in the purification of antibodies, enzymes and hormones (Cuacatrecasas and Anfinsen, 1970).

A prerequisite for preparation of the resin to be used in affinity chromatography is prior knowledge of a ligand which will specifically bind with the protein to be isolated. Studies of the inhibition kinetics of the enzyme $C1\bar{s}$ have described low molecular weight competitive inhibitiors with very low inhibition constants (Bing, 1969). It appeared that some of the better inhibitors such as alpha-phenylguanidine ($K_i = 5\cdot48 \times 10^{-4} M$) or benzamidine ($K_i = 6\cdot03 \times 10^{-4} M$) might be easily modified in order to provide functional groups for covalent linkage to a variety of resins. We have used meta-aminobenzamidine (m-ABA)*, a compound which is structurally related to benzamidine, to prepare an affinity chromatographic resin for purification of $C1\bar{s}$. With this resin we have found it possible to prepare in a single step 20–30 mg of highly purified $C1\bar{s}$ from 200 ml of serum. Characterization of the $C1\bar{s}$ prepared by affinity chromatography indicated it exhibits the same type of heterogeneity described by Nagaki and Stroud (1970), e.g. there are two electrophoretically distinct forms of $C1\bar{s}$, one being a degradative product of the other.

EXPERIMENTAL

Materials and methods

Chemicals and reagents. All chemicals and solvents were reagent grade. Triple distilled water was used for all buffers. Meta-nitrobenzamidine was purchased from Aldrich Chemicals. Triton X-100 was obtained from Rohm and Haas Co., Philadelphia. Hemolysin (titer = 1/3000) was obtained from Behring Diagnostics. C1 inactivator 1000 units/ml was obtained from Cordis Laboratories. Highly purified $C1\bar{s}$ was a gift from Dr. I. H. Lepow, Chairman, Department of Pathology, Health Center, University of Connecticut, Hartford, Conn. Sheep blood from a single male sheep, was collected into Alsever's solution and aged two weeks prior to use. Guinea pig blood was obtained by cardiac puncture from retired breeders donated by the Michigan State Public Health Laboratories. The blood was allowed to clot overnight at 4°C and the serum harvested by centrifugation at 2500 rev/min at 4°C. All complement components and sera were stored at −40°C.

Chemical procedures. Preparation of m-ABA—Sepharose: The procedure of Cuacatrecasas *et al.*(1968) was used to covalently link m-ABA to Sepharose. One hundred milliliters of settled Sepharose 6B (Pharmacia Fine Chemicals) was mixed with 100 ml of H_2O. Ten grams of CNBr (Eastman Organic Chemicals) in 200 ml of H_2O was added to the resin and the pH maintained at 11 by addition of $4 N$ NaOH with stirring until the pH remained constant (about 10 to 15 min). The Sepharose was washed with 2 l. of ice cold $0\cdot1 M$ NaH_2CO_3, pH 9·0, on a

---

*Abbreviations used include: m-ABA—meta-aminobenzamidine; N-Z-L-Tyr-p-Np—N-carbobenzoxy-L-tyrosine-para-nitrophenyl ester; N-A-L-Tyr-Et—N-acetyl-L-tyrosine-ethyl ester; EDTA—ethylenediaminetetraacetic acid; VBS—veronal buffered saline.

Buchner funnel with suction. Coupling of m-ABA was accomplished by mixing the CNBr treated-0·1 M NaH_2CO_3-washed Sepharose at 4°C with 5 g of m-ABA for 24 hr. Excess m-ABA was removed by filtration and washing on a Buchner funnel with suction. This procedure was repeated three times and the final m-ABA substituted Sepharose was mixed with an equal volume of untreated Sepharose 6B to increase the flow rate of the resin. The coupled material was stored at 4°C in H_2O with 0·005 M sodium azide until used.

Preparation of m-ABA: Five grams of meta-nitrobenzamidine · HCl (Aldrich Chemicals) dissolved in 200 ml of ethanol and 50 ml of H_2O was reduced at 40 psi of H_2 with 200 mg of 5 per cent Palladium of Charcoal as a catalyst in a Parr Hydrogenation apparatus. The catalyst was removed by filtration and the material concentrated to a syrup at 35 to 40°C in a Flash Evaporator (Buchner Instruments). The hydrochloride salt formed upon the addition of concentrated HCl. Recrystallization yielded 3 grams of meta-aminobenzamidine · HCl, m.p. = 279 to 281°C. The infrared spectrum (KBr pellet) indicated γ_{max} (cm^{-1}) 1675 (C = NH imine) and 1520 (C = NH imine). the m-ABA was stored at −20°C until used.

Immunochemical procedures. Immunoelectrophoresis was performed using a micro-modification of the procedure described by Scheidegger (1955), with the Gelman apparatus (Gelman Instruments). The agar for immunodiffusion and immunoelectrophoresis (Ion Agar, Difco) was made at a concentration of 1 per cent in 0·025 μ Tris-Barbital EDTA buffer, pH 8·9 (Williams and Chase, 1968). The immunoelectrophoresis and immunodiffusion plates were incubated over-night at room temperature and then for one week at 0°C. They were examined daily for a week to detect any secondary precipitin lines which might appear. Twenty-five to fifty microliters of antiserum were used to develop immuno-electrophoresis slides and gel diffusion plates.

Antiserum was raised in New Zealand white albino rabbits (Mr. D. Dillingham, Dewitt, Michigan) using the following immunization schedule: one mg of protein emulsified in complete Freund's adjuvant (BBL Laboratories) was injected into each hind foot pad and into 4 additional sites subcutaneously along the back. Each rabbit thus received a total of 6 mg of protein upon the initial immunization. Three weeks later, they were boosted with 2 mg of alum precipitated protein injected intraperitoneally. The animals were bled 6 days after the last injection, and serum collected after allowing the blood to clot overnight at 4°C. All antisera were inactivated at 56°C and absorbed with 1 ml of 50 per cent EA per 10 ml of serum prior to use.

The hemolytic activity of $C1\bar{s}$ was measured using a modification of the procedure described by Lepow *et al.* (1963). One tenth of a milliliter of various dilutions of $C1\bar{s}$ was mixed with 0·5 ml of EAC4, 1×10^8 cells/ml, (Borsos and Rapp, 1963), and 2·4 ml of guinea pig complement diluted 1:20 in VBS containing $1·5 \times 10^{-2} M$ MgEDTA. The mixtures were shaken at 30°C for 30 min and then incubated at 37°C for 60 min. The tubes were centrifuged, 2 ml of 0·15 M NaCl added and the extinctions read at 410 nm. Effective molecules/ml were calculated according to the method described by Borsos and Rapp (1963). Controls included EAC4 and C MgEDTA in the absence of $C1\bar{s}$ and $C1\bar{s}$ and EAC4 in the absence of C MgEDTA. The extent of hemolysis was determined by comparison to 0·5 ml of EAC4 lysed with 2·5 ml of a 1:100 dilution of guinea pig serum. Functionally pure guinea pig C1 was prepared according to methods described by Nelson *et al.* (1966) and contained 3×10^{10} effective molecules per ml (Borsos and Rapp, 1963).

Analytical procedures. Discontinuous acrylamide electrophoresis was performed with the vertical gel electrophoresis apparatus (E.C. Corporation, Philadelphia, Pa.). The stacking and running gels were prepared and electrophoresis was run according to directions supplied with the apparatus. A voltage of 7 V/cm was applied and electrophoresis was allowed to proceed until the tracking dye had moved 8–9 cm from the origin. Bands were located by staining with 0·25 per cent amido black dissolved in methanol, water, glacial acetic acid (5:5:1, v/v/v). The gel was destained by allowing it to stand in 7 per cent acetic acid.

Infrared spectra were obtained with a Perkin Elmer IR 700 Spectrometer. The samples were dried and prepared as KBr pellets using 1 mg of sample per 200 mg of KBr.

A Shimadzu-Double 40 u.v.-visible spectrophotometer was used for all enzymatic assays as well as for routine determination of absorbancy at other wave lengths.

Zonal electrophoresis was performed at pH 8·6 in 0·05 μ Barbital buffer (Williams and Chase, 1968) on a block of Pevikon (Pevikon C870, Stockholms Superfosfat fabriks A-B, Stockholm, Sweden) 15·5 cm × 38·5 cm × 1 cm. Pevikon was prepared as previously described (Manni and Müller-Eberhard, 1969). The protein was applied 14 cm from the cathode and electrophoresed for 16 hr at 10 V/cm. One centimeter strips were cut and eluted with 0·05 μ Barbital buffer, pH 8·6. Protein was located using the procedure of Lowry *et al.* (1951). The enzyme activity was measured using the substrate N-A-L-Tyr-Et.

Isolation of the euglobulin fraction of serum. The euglobulin fraction of serum was isolated by precipitation at an ionic strength of 0·02 and pH of 5·5 (Lepow *et al.*, 1963). The precipitate was dissolved at 0°C with stirring in a volume of 0·5 M NaCl equal to one tenth of the original volume of serum. It was dialyzed 18 hr at 4°C against two 2-l. changes of 0·15 μ sodium phosphate buffer, pH 7·4 (Haines and Lepow, 1964) activated at 37°C for 15 min, and then dialyzed 18 hr at 4°C against two 2-l. changes of 0·02 μ sodium phosphate buffer, pH 6·3 (Williams and Chase, 1968), containing 0·1 M NaCl and $1 \times 10^{-3} M$ Na$_2$H$_2$EDTA. The protein was centrifuged 1 hr at 15,000 rev/min prior to application to the column. Precipitated protein was washed one time with 5–10 ml of 0·02 μ sodium phosphate buffer containing 0·1 M NaCl $- 1 \times 10^{-3} M$ EDTA, and this was combined with the supernatant to yield the fraction of serum designated E.

Chromatography of euglobulin fraction on m-ABA—Sepharose. A 1·2 × 20 cm column of the m-ABA—Sepharose was poured and equilibrated at 4°C with 0·02 μ NaPO$_4$ buffer, pH 6·3, containing 0·1 M NaCl and $1 \times 10^{-3} M$ Na$_2$H$_2$EDTA, until the pH and conductivity of the effluent was identical to the equilibration buffer. Twenty milliliters of the euglobulin fraction of serum, dialyzed for 24 hr at 4°C against 3 changes of 2 l. of the equilibration buffer, were applied to the column, and 5 ml fractions collected. The column was washed at 4°C with the same buffer until the extinction at 280 nm (fraction 1) of the effluent was less than 0·050. The column was then eluted with 0·1 M propanoic acid, until the extinction at 280 nm was less than 0·050 (fraction 2). The column was finally eluted with

0·1 M acetic acid (fraction 3). To regenerate the column, about 200 ml of 0·1 M NaOH was washed through the column, and then the column reequilibrated against the 0·02 μ Na phosphate buffer, pH 6·3, containing 0·1 M NaCl and 1 × $10^{-3} M$ EDTA. Tubes containing protein were pooled, dialyzed immediately against cold 0·15 μ Na phosphate buffer, pH 7·4 (Haines and Lepow, 1964), and concentrated to about 10 ml in an Amicon Diaflo concentrator using a UM 10 membrane. They were stored at −40°C until used.

Enzyme assays. All substrates were recrystallized 2 times before use. The assay for hydrolysis of N-A-L-Tyr-Et was done at 37°C in 1 ml volumes. The micro-formol titration procedure was used to measure acid released (Levey and Lepow, 1959). The total amount of acid released was corrected for a blank containing only buffer, and calculated as μ moles of acid formed per ml of protein. One unit of enzyme was defined as that amount of protein which released a total of 0·5 μ moles of acid in 15 min at 37°C from 1 ml of $5 \times 10^{-3} M$ N-A-L-Tyr-Et. The assay for hydrolysis of N-Z-L-Tyr-p-Np was done at 25°C in 1·5 ml volumes containing $3 \times 10^{-5} M$ p-nitrophenyl-N-Z-L-Tyr (Bing, 1969). A tangent was drawn to the slope to obtain v, the initial rate of hydrolysis. One unit was defined as that amount of protein which produced 1×10^{-6} m-moles of para-nitrophenol in 5 min at 25°C at $5 \times 10^{-5} M$ N-Z-L-Tyr-p-Np.

To measure inhibition with C1 inactivator, the enzyme was preincubated 10 min at room temperature with indicated amounts of inactivator and then assayed for enzymatic activity using either of the above described procedures.

RESULTS

The separation of C1s̄ from the euglobulin fraction of serum was accomplished in a single step by chromatography on m-ABA − Sepharose (Fig. 1). Table 1 summarizes the results of two typical experiments. The euglobulin fraction was prepared and applied to the column as described in *Materials and Methods*. The majority of the protein applied was not adsorbed (fraction 1). Protein representing 5–6 per cent of the euglobulin fraction was eluted by the propanoic and acetic acids (fractions 2 and 3) (see Fig. 1). The protein recovery in the two experiments was 61 and 98 per cent for experiments A and B respectively. In experiment B, the resin was regenerated with 0·1 N NaOH after use in experiment A. It was noted that protein recoveries were always close to 100 per cent if the column had been previously saturated with protein.

All fractions had enzymatic activity towards N-A-L-Tyr-Et and N-Z-L-Tyr-p-Np. The increase in specific activity of fractions 2 and 3 was usually 10–20 times that of the euglobulin fraction. The specific activity of the enzyme was always slightly lower in fraction 3, probably indicating greater instability in the acetic acid. A comparable assay of highly purified C1s̄ obtained from Dr. I. H. Lepow is included for comparison (Table 1, experiment D).

Fractions 2 and 3 were not homogeneous when examined by acrylamide electrophoresis. Both contained at least 3 bands, a slow band, a fast band and a band migrating with the tracking dye (see arrows, Fig. 2A). Qualitative examination indicated fraction 2 was predominantly the slow band and fraction 3 contained both slow and fast bands in equal amounts. Fractions 2 and 3 each had a single precipitin band and complete reactions of identity in gel diffusion experi-

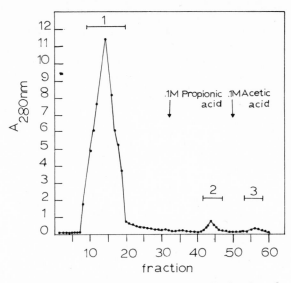

Fig. 1. Chromatography of the euglobulin fraction of serum on m-ABA—Sepharose. The arrows indicate the point of addition of $0 \cdot 1\,M$ propanoic and $0 \cdot 1\,M$ acetic acid.

ments with rabbit anti-human antiserum or rabbit antiserum to a mixture of fractions 2 and 3 (Figs. 2D, 2E). The two fractions were mixed and concentrated to 9·5 mg/ml and subjected to acrylamide electrophoresis. This concentrated material was composed of predominantly the faster migrating protein (Fig. 2A).

Immunoelectrophoresis of the concentrated mixture of fractions 2 and 3 and development with either rabbit anti-human serum antiserum or rabbit antiserum against the mixture of fractions 2 and 3 resulted in a fast (B) and a slow (A) migrating fraction both of which had enzymatic activity (Fig. 3).

The enzyme eluted from m-ABA—Sepharose by the dilute organic acids was identified as C1s̄ by the following experiments: First, the enzymatic activity, whether measured with N-A-L-Tyr-Et or N-Z-L-Tyr-p-Np, was tested for inhibition by C1 inactivator. In these experiments a saturating amount of C1 inactivator (50–100 units) was incubated 10 min with various amounts of enzyme prior to enzymatic assay. The composite results indicate that the enzyme in the acid fractions is completely inhibitable by C1 inactivator (Table 2).

Second, the enzyme was tested for a reaction of identity with anti-C1s̄ antiserum in gel diffusion experiments. A mixture of fraction 2 and fraction 3 (9·8 mg/ml) was reacted with antisera against C1s̄ and a mixture of 2 and 3. There was a line of identity within 10 hr. The second band with anti-C1s̄ appeared at about 36 hr (Fig. 2F).

Third, the protein caused the formation of E* in the presence of EAC4 and absence of a source of C̄1. The hemolysis of EAC4 was inhibitable by the anti-C1s̄ antiserum employed in the gel diffusion experiments (Table 3). The activity

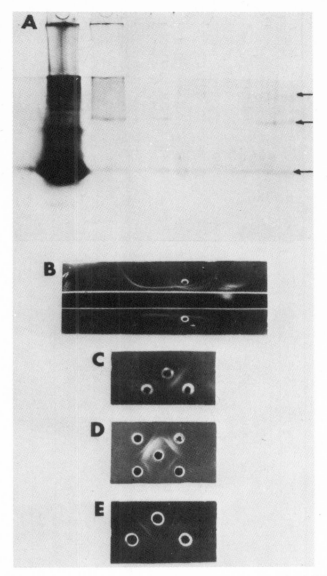

Fig. 2. Acrylamide electrophoresis, immunoelectrophoresis and gel diffusion experiments with fractions from m-ABA — Sepharose. A. Samples from left to right: whole serum, fraction E, 19 mg/ml; fraction 1, 5 mg/ml; fraction 2, 0·5 mg/ml, fraction 3, 0·7 mg/ml; and mixture of fraction 2 and 3, 9·8 mg/ml. B. Top well, whole serum; trough, anti-human serum antiserum; bottom well, mixture of fractions 2 and 3, 9·8 mg/ml. C. Center well, anti-mixture of fractions 2 and 3 antiserum; right well, fraction 3, 0·5 mg/ml; left well, fraction 2, 0·5 mg/ml. D. Samples clockwise: euglobulin, fraction 1, fraction 2, and fraction 3; center well, anti-human serum antiserum. E. Center well, mixture of fractions 2 and 3, 9·8 mg/ml; right well, anti-Cls̄-antiserum; left well, anti-mixture of fractions 2 and 3.

Table 1. Purification of Cls by chromatography on m-ABA – Sepharose

Exp. No.	Fraction	Volume (ml)	Protein (mg/ml)[a]	Protein Total	Enzyme activity N-A-L-Tyr-Et (units/ml)	N-A-L-Tyr-Et S.A.	N-A-L-Tyr-Et Total units	N-Z-L-Tyr-p-Np (units/ml)	N-Z-L-Tyr-p-Np S.A.	N-Z-L-Tyr-p-Np Total units
A	Serum	200								
	E	20	19·400	388·0	536	27·6	10,720	562	29·0	11,340
	1	72	2·950	212·0	174	29·5	12,510	264	79·0	19,000
	2	50	0·240	12·0	112	466·0	5600	139	590·0	6950
	3	43	0·337	14·5	117	347·0	5010	160	475·0	6880
B[b]	Serum	400								
	E	40	19·800	792·0	612	30·9	24,550	900	45·5	36,000
	1	130	4·100	738·0	60	14·6	10,800	86·5	21·1	15,600
	2	81	0·355	28·8	171	482·0	13,750	196	552·0	15,860
	3	85	0·127	10·8	47	370·0	3980	66	520·0	5600
C[c]	Serum									
	E	110	2·100	231·6				140	66·7	15,400
	1A	196	0·500	98·0				61	122·0	11,396
	1B	95	0·175	16·5				63	360·0	5960
D	Cls					502·0			612·0	

See *Results* for experimental details.

[a]The protein concentration was determined by using the method of Lowry *et al.* (1957). Bovine serum albumin was used as a standard.

[b]Experiment B is the combined results from 20 ml of E chromatographed simultaneously on two 1·2 × 20 cm columns.

[c]Experiment C is the results of recycling fraction 1 on m-ABA–Sepharose.

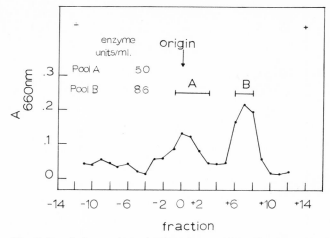

Fig. 3. Zonal electrophoresis of a mixture of fractions 2 and 3.
See *Materials and methods* for experimental details.

was not due to C$\overline{1}$; washing EAC4 treated with C1$\overline{s}$ prior to addition of C MgEDTA resulted in no hemolysis. According to this assay procedure, most preparations of C1$\overline{s}$ had between 2×10^9 and 4×10^9 effective molecules/mg of protein. The fact that, by all criteria, the enzyme eluted from the affinity chromatographic resin was C1$\overline{s}$ indicates that this material is probably the same as the two different molecular forms of C1$\overline{s}$ described by Nagaki and Stroud (1970).

More enzymatic activity was often recovered from the m-ABA — Sepharose than was applied. While this finding was reproducible the amount of activity

Table 2. Inhibition of fractions from m-ABA — Sepharose by Cl inactivator

Assayed with:	N-Z-L-Tyr-p-Np		N-A-L-Tyr-Et	
Fraction	Units of C1$\overline{s}$ without Cl inactivator	Units of C1$\overline{s}$ with Cl inactivator[a]	Units of C1$\overline{s}$ without Cl inactivator	Units of C1$\overline{s}$ with Cl inactivator[b]
E	1·80	0·80	1·65	0·20
	3·20	1·90	3·30	0·30
1	2·30	0·00	0·30	0·00
	4·65	0·03	0·90	0·00
2	2·50	0·00	4·90	0·00
	5·10	0·03	9·80	0·01
3	2·41	0·00	9·30	0·01
	4·90	0·00	6·60	0·02

See *Results* for experimental details.
[a]Fifty units of Cl inactivator were used.
[b]One hundred units of Cl inactivator were used.

recovered seemed to vary. The source of variation seemed to be in fraction 1; in fractions 2 and 3 the percentage of enzyme recovered as well as the specific activity of the enzyme was very consistent. The yield of Cl̄s protein was 5–6 per cent of that applied to the column and the specific activity was about 500 for N-A-L-Tyr-Et and 600 for N-Z-L-Tyr-p-Np. In contrast, it was found that total activity in fraction 1 could vary from containing activity equal to 1/2 to 2 times the total amount of enzyme applied to the column; the specific activity ranged from 20 to 70 for both substrates.

Table 3. Activity of Cl̄s in hemolysis of EAC4

Fraction	mg/ml	Effective molecules/ml		Effective molecules/mg protein
E	19·000		$4·63 \times 10^9$	$2·44 \times 10^9$
1	1·325	a	$6·08 \times 10^8$	$4·59 \times 10^8$
		b	0	
2	0·647	a	$2·69 \times 10^9$	$4·1 \times 10^9$
		b	0	
		c	0	
3	0·964	a	$2·48 \times 10^9$	$2·39 \times 10^9$
		b	0	
		c	0	

See *Results* for experimental details.
[a]EAC4 + C MgEDTA.
[b]EAC4 + C MgEDTA + 0·1 ml of anti Cl̄s antiserum.
[c]EAC4 + Fraction washed before adding C MgEDTA.

It appeared that the enzyme was being activated during chromatography of the euglobulin fraction on m-ABA—Sepharose. In an attempt to isolate this enzyme, fraction 1 was rechromatographed on m-ABA—Sepharose. It was possible to isolate about a third of the enzyme by rechromatography (Table 1, experiment C). The enzyme in fraction 1B was concentrated and analyzed similarly to fractions 2 and 3. It contained both slow and fast electrophoretically migrating material, and it was active in hemolysis of EAC4 with 4×10^9 effective molecules/mg of protein.

When preparations of the fractions eluted by acid from m-ABA—Sepharose were concentrated by pressure dialysis, protein was lost and specific activities were dramatically lowered. This apparently was due to aggregation of the protein as evidenced by the appearance of a white fine precipitate in the concentrated fractions. After several unsuccessful attempts at resolubilizing the material, it was found that dialysis of the concentrated fractions against buffer containing 0·01 per cent Triton X-100, a non-ionic detergent, seemed to partially resolubilize the material. Higher pH buffers were also partially effective, but no agent was as effective as the detergent in resolubilizing the precipitated protein. Results showing the effect of detergent on Cl̄s activity are shown in Table 4. The enzyme activity is 5–10 times higher in the presence of 0·01 per cent Triton X-100, as compared to the same buffer containing no Triton X-100, or a higher pH buffer.

Table 4. Effect of Triton detergent on Cl$\bar{\text{s}}$
activity

Fraction	(mg/ml)	Buffer[a]		
		A	B	C
2	0·647	570	0	45·0
3	0·964	180	0	17·9
2 & 3	9·680	930	330	233·0

See *Results* for experimental details.

[a]The enzyme was dialyzed against the following buffers:

A Buffer — 0·005 μ Tris-HCl, pH 8·1, containing 0·09 mM NaCl/ml and 0·1 per cent Triton v/v.

B Buffer — 0·005 μ Tris-HCl, pH 8·1, containing 0·09 mM NaCl/ml.

C Buffer — 0·02 μ glycine–NaOH, pH 9·0.

DISCUSSION

The application of the technique of affinity chromatography for purification of Cl$\bar{\text{s}}$ is a simple, reliable method for obtaining highly purified preparations of this complement protein. Technically, the procedure is less complicated than other methods which have been employed to purify complement proteins (Müller-Eberhard, 1968; Haines and Lepow, 1964). The m-ABA—Sepharose conjugate is stable and the resin used in this investigation has been used for 6 months with no apparent loss of specificity or capacity. On one occasion, 1 N NaOH destroyed the fractionating properties of m-ABA—Sepharose with respect to Cl$\bar{\text{s}}$.

The resin as prepared is essentially a weak cation exchange resin, since the benzamidine possesses a positive charge at neutral pH. To eliminate a certain amount of the potential ion exchange properties we use buffers at ionic strengths of greater than 0·1 and a pH of 6·3. We estimate that the capacity of the m-ABA—Sepharose for Cl$\bar{\text{s}}$ at an ionic strength of 0·12 and pH 6·3 at 4°C is about 1 mg/ml of settled resin. The resin thus has the same high capacity reported for other affinity chromatographic resins (Cuacatrecasas *et al.*, 1968; Cuacatrecasas, 1970; Cuacatrecasas and Anfinsen, 1970). The high binding capacity of the m-ABA-Sepharose for Cl$\bar{\text{s}}$ is further indicated by the fact that it required weak acids to effect elution of the protein. We find it difficult to use columns with bed volumes in excess of 50 ml. The use of larger columns dramatically reduces the recovery of total protein, as well as enzyme to less than 6 per cent (Bing, unpublished observations), probably because the ratio of resin to protein increases and secondary binding of non-specific protein can occur via an ion exchange mechanism. Using protein preparations with less than 3 mg/ml gives similar results; the low recovery of protein in the experiment in which fraction 1 was recycled (Table 1) is an example of protein loss upon chromatography of dilute protein solutions on m-ABA—Sepharose.

In principle it should have been possible to elute the enzyme with a competitive inhibitor. Our experience with such an elution procedure was uniformly unsuccessful. One to two per cent solutions of Cls̄ competitive inhibitors such as benzamidine or alpha-phenylquanidine eluted only a small portion of the adsorbed enzyme. Furthermore, after exhaustive dialysis of the eluted protein against the 0·15 μ sodium phosphate buffer, pH 7·4, to remove the bound inhibitor, there was little or no enzymatic activity (Bing, unpublished observations). In contrast the weak organic acids eluted the adsorbed protein quantitatively and yielded enzymatically active protein with specific activities comparable to Cls̄ prepared by ion exchange chromatographic procedures.

The results further substantiate that the substrate N-Z-L-Tyr-p-Np behaves similarly to N-A-L-Tyr-Et with respect to Cls̄. The enzyme activities are higher with the nitrophenyl ester, as noted in a previous study (Bing, 1969). Even in crude preparations, however, it appears that most of the enzyme activity towards N-Z-L-Tyr-p-Np is due to Cls̄ since Cl inactivator inhibits hydrolysis of the ester (Table 2).

The yields of enzyme eluted by acid are very reproducible; in the first cycle of chromatography, the combined propanoic and acetic acid fractions yielded 125–130 μg of protein per initial ml of serum. The protein is Cls̄ as evidenced by the following: First, the enzyme hydrolyzes N-A-L-Tyr-Et, a substrate which is reasonably specific for Cls̄. Second, the protein is active in catalyzing the formation of E* from EAC4; this activity is removed by washing prior to the addition of C2 through C9 or by specific anti-Cls̄ antiserum. Third, the enzymatic activity is totally inhibitable by Cl inactivator with both the N-Z-L-Tyr-p-Np and N-A-L-Tyr-Et substrates.

Quantitatively the yield of enzyme eluted by acid approaches the total amount of Cls̄ which is in serum according to immunochemical determinations (Müller-Eberhard, personal communication). The micro-heterogeneity of Cls̄ described by Nagaki and Stroud (1970) is also found in these preparations. Fraction 2 seems to be predominantly the slow form, but after concentration and mixing fractions, the predominant protein detected in acrylamide electrophoresis has the electrophoretic mobility of an alpha-globulin.

We find that Cls̄ purified by this method is comparable in terms of specific activity to Cls̄ purified by ion exchange chromatography on DEAE and TEAE cellulose (provided by Dr. I. H. Lepow; Table 1, experiment D). The enzyme is not, however, homogeneous. It exhibits the same type of micro-heterogeneity reported by Nagaki and Stroud (1970); reaction with one rabbit anti-Cls̄ antiserum (Fig. 2F) in a gel diffusion plate results in the appearance of a second precipitin band after approximately 36 hr on incubation. Homogeneous preparations of Cls̄ should be possible, however, by preparative electrophoretic procedures.

There are two observations which were totally unexpected and for which we can only suggest explanations. The effect of Triton X-100 on the protein was quite dramatic. While it has been reported that purified Cls̄ forms aggregates (Haines and Lepow, 1964; Müller-Eberhard, personal communication), the aggregation of the enzyme purified by affinity chromatography was even more apparent. Protein at a concentration of 5–4 mg/ml in 0·15 phosphate buffer, pH 7·4, would precipitate from solution on standing at 0°C. It is possible that the acid caused some change in the conformation on the protein which enhanced the aggregation in neutral buffers. In any case, the effect was reversible, since dialysis against detergent resolubilized the protein and increased the activity. Also, the total yield of enzyme activity was always greater than 100 per cent and often approached double the total activity applied. The mechanism by which this occurs is not entirely clear, but we hypothesize that the incubation at 37°C for 15 min did not fully activate the enzyme, and that final activation was accomplished by chromatography on m-ABA—Sepharose. According to this interpretation, previous estimations of the concentration of Cls in serum must be low, and perhaps the proenzyme form of Cls is not completely measurable by the immunochemical procedures employed to date. Experiments are now in progress to test this hypothesis.

Acknowledgements—The excellent technical assistance of Miss Sandra Spurlock is gratefully acknowledged. The gifts of anti-Cls antiserum and highly purified Cls by Dr. I. H. Lepow, Chairman, Department of Pathology, Health Center, University of Connecticut, Hartford, Conn., are also gratefully acknowledged.

REFERENCES

(1969) Bing D. H., *Biochemistry* 8, 4503.
(1963) Borsos T. and Rapp H. J., *J. Immun.* 91, 851.
(1968) Cuacatrecasas P., Wilcheck M. and Anfinsen C. B., *Proc. natn. Acad. Sci. U.S.A.* 61, 636.
(1970) Cuacatrecasas P., *J. biol. Chem.* 245, 3059.
(1970) Cuacatrecasas P. and Anfinsen C. B., Enzyme purification and related techniques, in *Methods in Enzymology*. Academic Press, N.Y. In press.
(1964) Haines A. L. and Lepow I. H., *J. Immun.* 93, 456.
(1963) Lepow I. H., Naff G., Todd E., Pensky J. and Hinz C., *J. exp. Med.* 117, 951.
(1959) Levey L. R. and Lepow I. H., *Proc. Soc. exp. Med.* 101, 608.
(1951) Lowry O. H., Rosebrough N. J., Farr A. L. and Randall R. J., *J. biol. Chem.* 193, 265.
(1969) Manni J. A. and Müller-Eberhard H. J., *J. exp. Med.* 130, 1143.
(1968) Müller-Eberhard J. J., in *Advances in Immunology* (Edited by Dixon Jr. F. J. and Kunkel H. G.), Vol. 8, p. 2. Academic Press, N.Y.
(1970) Nagaki K. and Stroud R. M., *J. Immun.* 105, 162.
(1966) Nelson R. A., Jensen J., Gigli I. and Tamura I., *Immunochemistry* 3, 111.
(1955) Scheidegger J. J., *Int. Archs. Allergy* 7, 103.
(1968) Shin H. S. and Mayer M. M., *Biochemistry* 7, 2991.
(1968) Williams C. A. and Chase M. W., in *Methods in Immunology and Immunochemistry*, *Vol. II*, p. 365. Academic Press, N.Y.

RESOLUTION OF THE FIRST COMPONENT OF GUINEA PIG COMPLEMENT INTO THREE SUBUNITS, C1q, C1r AND C1s, AND THEIR HYBRIDIZATION WITH HUMAN C1 SUBUNITS*

FELIX G. SASSANO, HARVEY R. COLTEN ,
TIBOR BORSOS and HERBERT J. RAPP

Abstract — Guinea pig C1 was resolved by chromatography into subunits C1q, C1r and C1s. These subunits recombined to form a hemolytically active C1 molecule. Each of these subunits is capable of forming hybrid C1 molecules with the appropriate subunits of human C1. A sedimentation constant of 12S was found for the recombined homologous human, guinea pig and hybrid C1 molecules.

The first component of complement (C1) of human and guinea pig sera is a macromolecule with an approximate sedimentation constant of 16–18 (Colten *et al.*, 1968; Naff *et al.*, 1964). Upon treatment with the chelating agent EDTA, human C1 dissociates into three subunits, designated C1q, C1r and C1s (Lepow *et al* , 1963). These subunits can be separated by chromatography and ultracentrifugation; when mixed together in the presence of Ca^{++}, the subunits recombine to form C1. From evidence obtained by absorption of guinea pig EDTA plasma with immune aggregates Barbaro (1963) suggested the existence of the 11S (C1q) subunit in guinea pig C1. Since then studies on the effect of EDTA on the structure of guinea pig C1 have not been made. However the results of studies on the effect of ionic strength on human and guinea pig C1, as well as similarities in their function, suggested that human and guinea pig C1 may have similar structures. The experiments on the effect of ionic strength on C1 were interpreted to mean that at high ionic strength both human and guinea pig C1 dissociated into subunits of approximately equal size (Colten *et al.*, 1968). The evidence suggested that these subunits were not identical with those obtained by treatment with EDTA.

We have investigated the effect of EDTA on the molecular characteristics of guinea pig C1. The results, reported in this paper, indicate that guinea pig C1 is composed of subunits similar to those obtained from human C1 by treat-

---

*A preliminary version of this paper was presented at the Federation Meeting, Chicago, 1971 (*Fedn Proc.* **30**, 472 Abs, 1971).

The terms and abbreviations used in this paper conform to the recommendations outlined in "Nomenclature of Complement", *Bull. Wld. Hlth Org.* **39**, 935 (1968); except that the bar over the C1 subunits was omitted since their state of activation was not known.

ment with EDTA. We also found human and guinea pig C1 subunits inter-changeable, i.e. a functionally active hybrid C1 molecule can be prepared by recombining guinea pig subunits with human subunits. The sedimentation constant of the recombined guinea pig, human and hybrid C1 molecules was approximately 12S.

MATERIALS AND METHODS

Source and preparation of reagents used in the titration of C1 and C1 sub-units and the method of titration of C1 have been described (Rapp and Borsos, 1970).

Titration of C1 *subunits.* Preliminary experiments indicated that the rate of recombination of the subunits in the fluid phase was highly concentration dependent. Therefore, the following procedure was adopted for the titration of C1q, C1r and C1s. Dilutions of the subunit to be titrated were mixed with a large excess of the other two subunits in VBS–sucrose buffer ($\mu = 0.065$). The mixtures were incubated for 60 min at 30°C and at that time dilutions were made in VBS–sucrose buffer and the amount of C1 activity generated was determined with the standard hemolytic assay for C1. In some instances C1s activity was determined by mixing a stable cell intermediate EAC1q4 with dilutions of C1s in VBS sucrose buffer followed by incubation for 30 min at 30°C. Activated C1s reacted with EAC1q4 without the addition of C1r. The cells were lysed by the successive addition of guinea pig C2 and C-EDTA as in the hemolytic assay for C1. EAC1q4 were prepared by mixing EAC4 with a dilution of C1q (at least 50 effective C1q molecules/cell) in VBS–sucrose buffer ($\mu = 0.065$). The cells were incubated for 15 min at 30°C and were washed twice and resuspended in VBS–sucrose buffer to a concentration of 1.5×10^8 cells/ml.

Density gradients for ultracentrifugation of C1 and its subunits were pre-pared as described in (Colten *et al.*, 1968). In these studies an L2-65 ultracentri-fuge was used with a Spinco SW 39 rotor. In each experiment one centrifuge tube contained one or more of the following protein markers: thyroglobulin, rabbit IgG and bovine serum albumin. Sedimentation constants were estimated by the method of Martin and Ames (1961).

RESULTS AND DISCUSSION

The chromatographic separation of C1 *into subunits.* Human C1q, C1r and C1s were prepared by DEAE chromatography by the method of Lepow *et al.* (1963). The specificity of the subunits was confirmed with reagents kindly supplied by Dr. George B. Naff, Cleveland, Ohio. We then attempted to fractionate guinea pig C1 derived from a euglobulin precipitate ($\mu = 0.04$, pH 5.6) by the same method. Guinea pig C1 was separated into two fragments, one of which was similar to human C1q and the other presumably containing C1r and C1s, for this fraction generated C1 activity in the presence of human C1q. The two guinea pig C1 fragments also recombined to form hemolytically active C1.

In the next experiment a euglobulin precipitate of guinea pig serum was dialyzed overnight at 4°C against VBS saline containing 0.05M EDTA; this con-centration of EDTA represented a 50-fold increase in EDTA concentration over the amount used by Lepow *et al.* This euglobulin preparation was then chromatographed on DEAE as described by Lepow *et al.* The results of this experiment given in Fig. 1 show that guinea pig C1 was resolved into three fractions. The first fraction was identified as Clq for it was capable of generating Cl activity when mixed with human Clr and Cls. The second active fraction was like human Clr for it generated Cl activity when mixed with human Clq and Cls. The third peak of activity was identified as Cls by its reactivity with the human subunits Clq and Clr. In addition, the fractions designated as guinea pig Clq, Clr and Cls were capable of recombining to form a hemolytically active guinea pig C1 molecule. The results of the hemolytic titration of the recombined subunits are shown in Table 1. The major point emerging from these data is that hemolytically active C1 can be constructed from one or more subunits of one species with the complementary subunits of the other species. The hemolytic activity of these hybrid C1 subunits was also detected by their ability to lead to lysis of EA following addition of purified C4, C2 and C-EDTA.

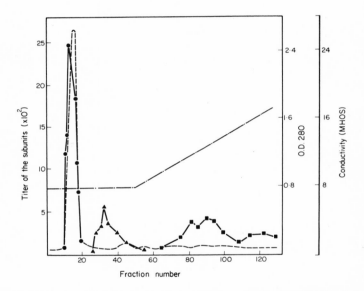

Fig. 1. Resolution of guinea pig C1 into three subunits by DEAE-cellulose chromatography. Clq (●), Clr (▲) and Cls (■). Optical density at 280 nm (– – –). Conductivity of elutrient (—·—·).

Ultracentrifugation of C1 *subunits.* Figures 2a, b and c show the results of ultracentrifugation of the subunits of guinea pig C1 and the marker proteins BSA, thyroglobulin and IgG. The sedimentation constant of guinea pig Clq was about 10·2–10·7, of Clr about 6·9–7·3 and of Cls about 4·3. These values are similar to those obtained for the human subunits (Naff *et al.*, 1964). Figure 3 shows the results of ultracentrifugation of homologous recombined human C1 and a hybrid C1 made from guinea pig Clq, and human Clr and Cls. Both C1 molecules have a sedimentation constant of about 12S.

Table 1. Hemolytic activity of recombined guinea pig (G) and human (H) Cl subunits

Guinea pig				Human				Hybrid			
q	r	s	Cl[a]	q	r	s	Cl	q	r	s	Cl
G	—	—	6	—	H	H	32	G	H	H	204
—	G	—	15	H	—	H	253	H	G	H	352
—	—	G	17	H	H	—	10	H	H	G	483
G	G	—	42	—	—	H	10	G	G	H	179
G	—	G	13	—	H	—	7	G	H	G	143
—	G	G	24	H	—	—	8	H	G	G	120
G	G	G	231	H	H	H	737				

[a]Reciprocal dilution of Cl yielding one effective Cl molecule/ml/cell.

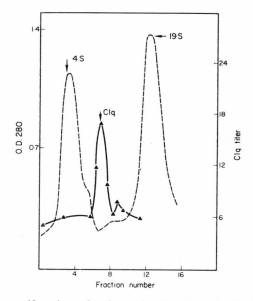

Fig. 2a. Ultracentrifugation of guinea pig Clq in veronal buffered saline $\mu = 0.15$ in a 10–28% sucrose gradient (at 10°C for 16 hr at 32,000 rev/min). Protein markers (– – –) at O.D. 280 nm. Bovine serum albumin = 4S, thyroglobulin = 19S and Clq (△). Fraction 1 = top of centrifuge tube.

The sedimentation constants of the recombined guinea pig and human subunits and of some of the recombined hybrid molecules were also determined. These results are summarized in Table 2.

The most important information emerging from this experiment is that the reconstituted Cl molecule (hybrid or homologous) had a sedimentation constant considerably lower than the intact Cl molecule. The results presented in Fig. 4 show that the lower S values could not be ascribed to the treatment of Cl with EDTA alone.

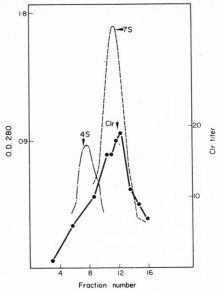

Fig. 2b. Ultracentrifugation of guinea pig C1r in veronal buffered saline $\mu = 0\cdot15$ in a 5–20% sucrose gradient (at 10°C for 23 hr at 38,000 rev/min). Protein markers $(\cdot\!-\!\cdot) =$ BSA (4S) and $(-\,-\,-) =$ IgG (7S) at O.D. 280 nm. C1r $= (\bullet)$. Fraction 1 $=$ top of centrifuge tube.

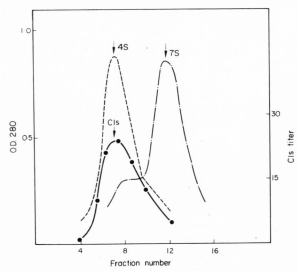

Fig. 2c. Ultracentrifugation of guinea pig C1s in veronal buffered saline $\mu = 0\cdot15$ in a 5–20% sucrose gradient (at 10°C for 22 hr at 38,000 rev/min). Protein markers at O.D. 280 nm $(-\,-\,-)$ 4S $=$ BSA and $(\cdot\!-\!\cdot)$ 7S $=$ IgG. $(\bullet) =$ C1s. Fraction 1 $=$ top of centrifuge tube.

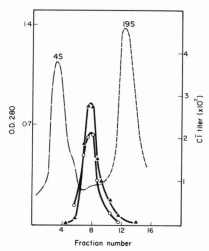

Fig. 3. Ultracentrifugation of homologous and hybrid forms of C1 (at 10°C for 16 hr at 32,000 rev/min). Hybrid C1 (▲) = gp C1q, hu C1r and hu C1s. Homologous C1 (●) = human C1qrs. Sucrose gradient 10–29% in VBS, $\mu = 0.15$. Protein markers (O.D. 280 nm) BSA (·—·) and thyroglobulin (- - -). Fraction 1 = top of centrifuge tube.

Table 2. Sedimentation constants of C1 hybrids

C1q^{gp}	C1r^{gp}	C1s^{gp}	12·7
C1q^{hu}	C1r^{hu}	C1s^{hu}	12·0
C1q^{gp}	C1r^{gp}	C1s^{hu}	10·0
C1q^{gp}	C1r^{hu}	C1s^{hu}	11·9
C1q^{hu}	C1r^{gp}	C1s^{hu}	13·6
C1q^{hu}	C1r^{hu}	C1s^{gp}	12·7

The following points emerge from these studies:

(1) Guinea pig C1 on treatment with EDTA followed by DEAE chromatography can be resolved into three subunits like those described for human C1 (Lepow *et al.*, 1963). However, we found it necessary to treat guinea pig C1 with 0·05 M EDTA to be able to resolve it into its subunits by chromatography.

(2) Hybrid C1 molecules could be prepared from the appropriate combination of the human and guinea pig subunits.

(3) When homologous guinea pig subunits or homologous human subunits were recombined or when guinea pig subunits were recombined with human subunits generating hybrid C1 molecules, the resultant hemolytically active C1 molecule had a sedimentation constant of about 12S ($\mu = 0.15$). An S value of 16–18 was obtained, however, for purified guinea pig C1, for C1 in guinea pig euglobulin and for C1 in guinea pig euglobulin dialyzed against EDTA with subsequent removal of EDTA. The lower sedimentation constant (12S) for recombined C1qrs suggested two possibilities: (a) the C1 molecule generated

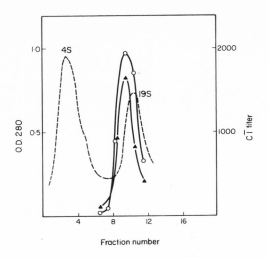

Fig. 4. Ultracentrifugation of guinea pig Cl in euglobulin treated with EDTA.
EDTA removed by dialysis against VBS, $\mu = 0\cdot065$ containing Ca^{++} and Mg^{++}.
Sucrose gradient 10–28% in VBS, $\mu = 0\cdot15$; temperature $= 10°C$; time $= 16$
hr; 32,000 rev/min. (○) Euglobulin dialyzed against VBS, $\mu = 0\cdot15$ containing
Ca^{++} and Mg^{++}. (▲) Euglobulin dialyzed against VBS, $\mu = 0\cdot15$ with $0\cdot05\,M$
EDTA then against VBS, $\mu = 0\cdot065$ containing Ca^{++} and Mg^{++}. Optical
density (280 nm) $=$ protein markers (– – –), $4S = BSA$ and $19S =$ thyroglobulin.
Fraction 1 $=$ top of centrifuge tube.

from subunits has a shape different from the native Cl molecule, or (b) multiples
of one or more of the subunits are present in the native Cl and not all of them
are necessary for recombination. Evidence that human Cl contains more than
one Cls per Clq was presented recently (Müller-Eberhard, 1970).

One of the difficulties which was observed by Lepow (1963) and by us was that
after Cl was reconstructed from its subunits, not more than 20 per cent of the
original Cl activity could be accounted for. Exposure to the relatively high
concentration of EDTA before DEAE chromatography was considered to be a
possible source of low activity for the Cl in the reconstructed Cl preparations.
We therefore studied the effect of EDTA and its subsequent removal by dialysis
(in the presence of Ca^{++} and Mg^{++}) on the hemolytic activity of human and
guinea pig Cl. We found that the Cl present in whole serum was almost irrever-
sibly inactivated by $0\cdot05\,M$ EDTA while Cl purified by zonal ultracentrifugation
regained up to 50 per cent of its hemolytic activity upon removal of EDTA. Cl
present in a euglobulin fraction had an intermediate potential for reactivation.
Data supporting these conclusions are presented in Table 3. We can offer no
explanation for the differences in the behavior of Cl in whole serum, in
euglobulin and in highly purified form with respect to inactivation by
EDTA. However, it is possible that in whole serum proper recombination is
prevented by other serum constituents; these interfering substances may have
been removed during purification.

64

Table 3. Effect of EDTA and its subsequent removal on the hemolytic activity of C1

	VBS $\mu = 0.15$ EDTA $0.05\,M$ hours dialyzed					VBS–Sucrose $\mu = 0.065$ Ca^{++} $0.00015\,M$/Mg^{++} $0.001\,M$ hours dialyzed			
	0	0·5	2	6		0	3	8	21
GP serum	42,000	14,000	13,000	1600	→	2000	1500	3500	2000
GP C$\bar{1}$	19,000	1600	—	—	→	230	1500	4500	3200
Hu serum	112,000	42,000	31,000	14,000	→	14,000	23,000	17,000	11,000
Hu C$\bar{1}$[a]	34,000	1900	—	—	→	1200	15,000	20,000	12,000
GP Euglob	42,000	—	4000	—	→	—	—	21,000	—

[a] C$\bar{1}$ = Purified by zonal ultracentrifugation.

REFERENCES

Barbaro J. F. (1963) *Nature, Lond.* **199**, 819.
Colten H. R., Borsos T. and Rapp H. J. (1968) *J. Immun.* **100**, 808.
Lepow I. H., Naff G. B., Todd E. W., Pensky J. and Hinz C. F. (1963) *J. exp. Med.* **117**, 983.
Martin R. G. and Ames B. N. (1961) *J. biol. Chem.* **236**, 1372.
Müller-Eberhard H. J. (1970) *Abstracts of the Eighth International Congress of Biochemistry,* p. 321.
Naff G. B., Pensky J. and Lepow I. H. (1964) *J. exp. Med.* **119**, 593.
Rapp H. J. and Borsos T. (1970) *Molecular Basis of Complement Action,* Appleton-Century-Crofts, New York.

ADDITIONAL STUDIES ON HUMAN C5: DEVELOPMENT OF A MODIFIED PURIFICATION METHOD AND CHARACTERIZATION OF THE PURIFIED PRODUCT BY POLYACRYLAMIDE GEL ELECTROPHORESIS

U. R. NILSSON, R. H. TOMAR and F. B. TAYLOR, Jr.

Abstract — This paper reports on the purification and characterization of human C5.

1. A modified isolation technique has been elaborated allowing the isolation of highly purified C5 within 5–7 days in yields of 1–2 mg per 100 ml processed serum.

2. In the process of developing this new procedure the difficulty of removing a trace plasminogen–plasmin contaminant from C5 was recognized. The new procedure employs a technique which eliminates this contaminant, and which prevents activation of plasmin during isolation. Since plasmin was found to degrade C5 proteolytically, possible plasmin dependent degradation of C5 during preparation can now be prevented.

3. Polyacrylamide gel electrophoresis in the presence of sodium dodecyl sulfate was employed in the study of reduced C5: (a) two polypeptide chains were demonstrable; (b) the mean molecular weights of these chains were 83000 (80–87000) and 123000 (120–125000) respectively in three independent tests; (c) since the native C5 molecule appears to contain one of each of these chains, the molecular weight of the intact C5 molecule appears to be approximately 206000.

INTRODUCTION

The only purification method so far available for the isolation of human C5 in a degree of purity and in amounts adequate for chemical work, has been the one described by Nilsson and Müller-Eberhard in 1965 (Nilsson and Müller-Eberhard, 1965). An advantage with this isolation technique is that it allows the simultaneous preparation of C3 as well as C5. A disadvantage is that it is relatively laborious and requires a long time for completion. In addition, the yield of C5 is relatively low.

Since our studies are concerned with C5 more than with C3, we felt prompted to develop an alternative, more time saving procedure for obtaining C5 in the pure form. This has now been accomplished by a rather extensive modification of the previously described method. In the process of developing this new isolation technique a trace plasminogen/plasmin (plg/pln)* contaminant of C5 prepared by the old method was recognized. The new method allows the removal of this contaminant. New information concerning the physical structure of C5 was gained during these studies in the analysis by polyacrylamide gel electrophoresis of isolated material.

*Abbreviations used: plg/pln = plasminogen/plasmin; SDS = sodium dodecyl sulfate; EACA = epsilon amino caproic acid; C = complement; C5 = fifth component of complement; MSH = mercaptoethanol.

MATERIALS AND METHODS

A. *Preparation and storage of C5*

Precipitation of a C5-rich euglobulin fraction from serum. Human blood collected without anti-coagulants was left at room temperature for approximately 2 hr to allow clotting and clot retraction to take place. Then the blood specimens were centrifuged for 30 min at 1600 **g** and 4°C. A few remaining red cells were removed from the subsequently decanted serum by an additional centrifugation under the same conditions. The serum was then used for C5 preparation either immediately or after freezing and storage at − 70°C in carefully sealed glass bottles. Rapid freezing of the serum was accomplished in a dry ice acetone bath.

A euglobulin precipitate rich in C5 was obtained from fresh or previously frozen and thawed human serum by dilution and acidification. The procedure was performed strictly at 4°C for its entire length. Serum was first diluted 3·7 times by adding 270 ml of 0·11 M l-lysine HCl to 100 ml of serum. The ionic strength of the l-lysine serum mixture was then lowered by the addition of distilled water (approximately 146 ml). After a conductance of 4·1 m-mho (measured at 4°C) was reached, the pH was adjusted to 5·0 by the addition of 1 M acetic acid (approximately 7·5 ml). The euglobulin precipitate formed during 3·5 hr of continuous magnetic stirring was sedimented by centrifugation at 8700 **g** for 15 min. The supernatant fluid was removed, and the precipitate washed by resuspension and sedimentation under similar conditions in three changes of washing solution which was prepared as follows. One volume saline was added to 2·7 volumes of 0·11 M l-lysine HCl. The mixture was diluted with H_2O to adjust the conductance to 4·1. Then the pH was lowered to 5·0 by the addition of 1 M acetic acid. After washing, the precipitate was dissolved in 0·03 M sodium PO_4 at a pH of 7·0 containing 0·1 M epsilon amino caproic acid (EACA).

Chromatographic procedures. The euglobulin fraction was directly applied to a 200 ml TEAE cellulose (Schleicher & Schuell, Lot no. 1919, 0·88 m-equiv./g dry weight) column (i.d., 2·5 and length 40 cm) packed by hydrostatic pressure and previously equilibrated with 0·03 M PO_4 buffer at a pH of 7·0, containing 0·1 M EACA with a conductance of 2·5 m-mho (starting buffer). The column was eluted by gradually increasing the NaCl concentration in the eluting buffer. Two 1-l. beakers connected by a siphon were used as a gradient making device. The beaker serving as the mixing chamber was initially filled with starting buffer and the other with the similar buffer to which NaCl had been added to give a conductance of 9·0 m-mho at 4°C (= limiting buffer). The column eluate which was collected in 15 ml fractions by the use of an automatic fraction collector was analyzed by the Folin method (protein) by a semi-quantitative double diffusion technique as described by Nilsson and Müller-Eberhard (1965), and by the C5 hemolytic assay technique. Fractions containing C5 were pooled and further processed by hydroxyl apatite chromatography.

Commercially available hydroxyl apatite (Bio-Rad's hydroxyl apatite for chromatography, Biogel HT, contr No. 9149, Date 8/24/70) prepared by the method of Tiselius *et al.* (1956) was used. The columns were packed by hydrostatic pressure in glass tubes with an i.d. of 2 cm. The size of the OH apatite column was determined by the amount of protein that was going to be separated.

The ratio of protein (mg):volume (ml) of packed OH apatite was kept at 1·2. Before application to the OH apatite column, the conductance of the C5 containing pool was adjusted to 3 m-mho (at 4°C) by the addition of 0·1 M EACA in distilled H_2O. It was then applied to the column without any preceding concentration procedure or pH adjustment. The column was equilibrated with an EACA-containing (0·1 M) sodium potassium PO_4 buffer of a pH of 7·9 and of a conductance of 3 m-mho at 4°C (5 m-mho at 23°C), (starting buffer). The column was eluted by gradually increasing the PO_4 concentration in the eluting buffer. Two 200 ml beakers, connected with a siphon, were used as the gradient making device. The beaker serving as a mixing chamber was initially filled with starting buffer. The other beaker was filled with an EACA-containing (0·1 M), sodium potassium PO_4 buffer of a concentration giving a conductance of 15·5 m-mho at 4°C (25 m-mho at 23°C) (limiting buffer). The gradient elution was started immediately after the application of the protein to the column was completed. Buffers used for OH apatite chromatography were prepared from 0·02 M sodium PO_4 buffer (Buffer No. 1) and 0·65 M sodium-potassium PO_4 buffer (Buffer No. 2), both of which had a pH of 7·9 and contained 0·1 M EACA. By mixing buffer No. 1 and No. 2 mixtures of the desired PO_4 concentration, as gauged by conductance measurements were obtained. Buffer No. 2 was obtained by adjusting the pH of a 0·65 M K_2H PO_4 to 7·9 by adding 0·65 M NaH_2 PO_4. The column eluate collected in 2 ml fractions was analyzed by the same procedure as those employed for the eluate obtained by TEAE cellulose chromatography.

Procedures employed for the concentration and storage of purified C5. Fractions of human C5 purified by OH apatite chromatography were concentration in an Amicon concentration device Model No. 12 by positive pressure filtration through PM30 filters (Amicon). Preparations ranging in concentration from 0·2 to 3·0 mg/ml were dialyzed vs. PO_4, pH 7, μ 0·1, with or without 0·1 M EACA added and subsequently frozen in dry ice acetone in small aliquots, which were kept in well-sealed vials at $-70°$ until used.

B. *Analysis of C5*

Treatment of C5 with reducing and alkylating agents. The effect of mercaptoethanol (MSH) on purified C5 was studied, (a) when C5 was first treated with MSH, and subsequently alkylated with iodoacetamide, or (b) when C5 was treated with MSH, and subsequently maintained in the reduced state in excess MSH.

All procedures involved in condition (a) were performed under N_2 gas with solutions that had previously been evacuated 2× and equilibrated with N_2 gas. Routinely, 30 μg C5 in 10 μl PO_4, pH 7·0, μ 0·1 was mixed with 10 μl of a 0·115 M glycine solution, pH 10·0 (glycine buffer) and 5 μl MSH solution in glycine buffer. The concentration of the MSH solution was 5× that desired in the final 25 μl reaction volume. After 30 min incubation at room temperature, 50 μl glycine buffer containing iodoacetamide in 10× molar excess to the previously added MSH. After an additional 30 min incubation at room temperature, the test material was made up to 200 μl with PO_4 buffer, pH 7·0, μ 0·1 and incubated at 37°C for 2 hr in 1% SDS as described below and subsequently analyzed by polyacrylamide gel electrophoresis.

Reduction of C5 under condition (b) was performed in a modification of

Weber and Osborn's procedure (1969). Thirty μg of C5 in PO$_4$ buffer, pH 7·0, μ 0·1 were incubated for 2 hr at 37°C in the presence of 1% sodium dodecyl sulfate (SDS) (w/v) and 1% mercaptoethanol (volume 14M stock solution per volume reaction mixture). The whole reaction mixture (0·2 ml) plus 5 lambda additional 14M MSH were analyzed by polyacrylamide gel electrophoresis, without preceding dialysis (see below). Proteins used as molecular weight markers were treated in an identical manner.

Gel filtration. Gel filtration analysis of purified C5 was performed at room temperature on a Sepharose 6B (Pharmacia), column (bed vol = 142 ml, 1·5 cm × 80 cm) equilibrated with veronal buffered saline (Mayer, 1961) containing 0·1% sodium dodecyl sulfate (SDS). A mixture of ^{125}I-labelled (6%) and non-labelled (94%) purified C5 was analyzed either in the non-reduced state or after reduction and alkylation as described below. Test material analyzed by gel filtration under these conditions was first incubated in a 1% SDS solution for 2 hr, and then in an ice bath for 2–3 hr. The soluble portion of the sample which contained the bulk of the protein was removed from the insoluble portion of the SDS which precipitated in the cold as crystals. The sample was mixed with Blue Dextran and then applied to the column.

The column eluate was collected in 1·5 ml fractions which were analyzed for their content of Blue Dextran (OD 635), ^{125}I counts and protein (OD$_{210}$).

Polyacrylamide gel electrophoresis. Polyacrylamide gel electrophoresis analysis was performed under two conditions: (a) in a basic buffer system, as described by Davis (1964), or (b) in a basic buffer system, in the presence of a 0·1% sodium dodecyl sulfate (SDS) as described by Weber and Osborn (1969).

When the analysis was performed under condition (a) running gels of 5% and spacer gels of 3% polyacrylamide concentrations were used. Under condition (b) the polyacrylamide concentrations of the corresponding gels were 7·5 and 3% respectively. Under both conditions an amperage of 4–5 mA/gel was employed. Electrophoresis for each individual gel was interrupted when the Bromphenol blue tracking dye had reached the anodal end of the gel. Bromphenol blue was present in 0·1% concentration in the buffer of the top buffer compartment of the electrophoresis apparatus.

Routinely 30 μg of C5 were applied in a volume of 200 μl if necessary adjusted by the addition of a phosphate buffer of a pH of 7·0 and a μ of 0·1. A few granules of sucrose and dry Sephadex G25 particles were also added in order to prevent loss by convection. Non-reduced C5 was analyzed in the absence of SDS (condition (a)) or in the presence of SDS (condition (b)) following preincubation of the test sample at 37°C for 2 hr with 1% SDS. Reduced or reduced and alkylated (see above) material was analyzed under condition (b). The following polypeptide molecular weight markers were employed when the method was applied to molecular weight determination of C5 (Weber and Osborn, 1969): Human Myosin kindly supplied by Dr. Audrey Penn, Dept. of Neurology, Univ. of Pa., Phila., Pa.; Phosphorylase-a from rabbit muscle purchased from Sigma, Lot No. 11C-0480; Human IgG purchased from Mann Research Laboratories, Lot No. 457; Human albumin purchased from Behringwerke, Batch 3708.

Following electrophoresis the gels were stained with the amido schwarz or with the coomassie brilliant blue dyes and subsequently destained electrophoretically or by washing respectively. Analysis for C5 was also performed by the Ouchterlony technique by the hemolytic assay procedure or by radioactivity counting when ^{125}I labelled C5 was studied. These procedures required that the gels were first sectioned into 1 or 2 mm segments, which was accomplished with the aid of a template and a razor blade. When C5 was determined by the Ouchterlony technique (according to Hayward and Augustin's, 1957) the cut polyacrylamide gel sgements were fused into an agarose slide. A monospecific anti-C5 antiserum was used to develop the immunodiffusion patterns. Hemolytic analysis for C5 was performed on eluates obtained from crushed gel segments kept at 4°C overnight in 0·5 ml veronal buffered saline (Mayer, 1961) containing 0·1% gelatin.

Immunodiffusion techniques. Antisera of the following specificity and origin were utilized for the immunochemical analysis.

Anti whole human serum — (Rabbit) Behring Diagnostics, Inc., Division of American Hoechst Corporation, Somerville, N.J., Batch No. 1704F and 1586y

Anti human plasmin — (Rabbit) Behring Diagnostics, Inc., Batch No. 1996 Anti human Ig antiserum with specificity for IgG, IgA and IgM — (Rabbit) Behring Diagnostics, Inc., Batch No. 1677B.

Anti human $\beta1H$ — (Rabbit) prepared as described by Nilsson and Müller-Eberhard (1965).

Anti human C4 — (Rabbit) kindly donated by Dr. Müller-Eberhard *et al.*

Anti human C3 — (Rabbit) prepared as described by Nilsson and Müller-Eberhard (1965).

Anti human C5 — (Rabbit and mouse) prepared as described by Nilsson and Müller-Eberhard (1965 and 1967).

Anti human C5 — (Goat) kindly donated by Dr. Müller-Eberhard *et al.*

The radial diffusion technique according to Mancini *et al.* (1964) was utilized for the quantitation of C3, C5 and plasminogen. Commercially available plates for radial diffusion were employed for the determination of C3 (Hyland Laboratories, Costa Mesa, Calif., Immunoplate, human complenent C3 test, list no. 085-150). C5 and plasminogen were quantitated in plates containing monospecific rabbit antiserum to human C5 or to human plasminogen incorporated in 1% agarose made up in veronal buffer, pH 8·6, μ 0·05, containing 0·01 M EDTA.

The Ouchterlony technique was employed for qualitative analysis and for semiquantitative analysis as described previously (Nilsson and Müller-Eberhard, 1965) or as described by Hayward and Augustin (1957).

Immunoelectrophoresis was performed on microscopic slides according to Scheidegger (1955).

Fibrinolytic assay for plgn/pln. Plgn/pln was assayed for functionally by a fibrin plate assay technique previously described by Tomar and Taylor (1971). Fibrin plates were prepared by pouring 10 ml sodium PO_4 buffer at pH 7·4 and μ 0·087 containing 1·5% agar, 0·125% bovine fibrinogen and 3 U. of thrombin into a disposable petri dish of 10 cm diameter. Test material and streptokinase (2000 u SK/ml of Lederle's streptokinase–streptodornase in the same PO_4

buffer), were first mixed in equal aliquots. Three mm wide wells punched into the fibrin–agar plate were filled with the test mixture. After 24 hr incubation at room temperature, the zones of fibrinolysis around wells containing test material were measured and compared with those caused by dilutions of a standard human plasmin preparation. A linear relationship between area of fibrinolysis and log plgn/pln concentration was found with the standard material in a concentration range from 0·1–100 μg plg/pln per ml. The standard material was a purified plg/pln preparation in 50% glycerol made by G. Sgouris for NIH, Div. of Biological Standards. It contained 10 Remmert and Cohen caseinolytic units per ml which approximately corresponds 0·3 mg plasmin per ml.

Hemolytic assay procedure for human C5. 'Molecular titration' of C5 in the isolated form and in whole human serum was performed by a modification by Nilsson and Miller (1971) of the procedure described by Cooper and Müller-Eberhard (1970). C5 was incubated at 30°C with sheep erythrocytes antibody complement intermediates in the EAC14^{oxy}23 state. After 10 min incubation a source of C6–C9 prepared from guinea pig serum was added and the cells were incubated an additional period of 60 min at 30°C. Hemolysis, measured spectrophotometrically and expressed as the average number of hits/cell, was found to vary in a linear fashion with the dose of added C5 in a range from 0 to 5 ng.

Protein determinations. Protein was determined by a modification of the Folin method (Kunkel, 1951). A standard curve relating OD_{700} and C5 protein, was constructed on the basis of a nitrogen (N) analysis, and an assumed conversion factor of C5 N to C5 protein = 6·25.

Radiolabelling of C5. Stroud's modification (1971) of the procedure of McConahey and Dixon (1966) was employed for the ^{125}I labelling of C5 with some alterations. Five-hundred μg of C5, 0·5 mc carrier free ^{125}I and 50 μg of Chloramin T (practical grade, J. T. Baker, Chem., lot no. 1-3517) in a total volume of 2 ml PO_4 buffer, pH 7·0, μ 0·1, were stirred at 4°C. After 5 min the sample was passed over a SX G25 coarse (Pharmacia) column, 1×50 cm equilibrated with the same PO_4 buffer, containing NaCl in a final concentration of 0·25 M. The C5 containing fractions of the eluate were dialyzed for 12 hr against a PO_4 buffer, pH 7·0 and μ 0·1 containing EACA at 0·1 M concentration, concentrated, frozen and stored at -70°C.

RESULTS

Demonstration of a plg/pln contaminant in preparations of C5, purified according to Nilsson and Müller-Eberhard (1965). Tests for plg/pln were performed on 10 different C5 preparations isolated according to Nilsson and Müller-Eberhard (1965) by the fibrinolytic assay procedure. All preparations showed fibrinolytic activity. Comparison of the activity of the different C5 preparations with that of dilutions of the standard plasmin preparation, indicated a level of plg/pln contamination ranging from 0·05 to 0·02% (w/w).

Enzymatic modification of C5 by plasmin. Fifty μg of C5 and 5 μg of plasmin in a final volume of 0·1 ml veronal buffered saline, pH 7·4 (Mayer, 1961) were incubated for 1 hr at 37°C. Fifty μg of C5 incubated at 37°C for the same time period in the absence of plasmin served as a control. Comparative analysis by immunoelectrophoresis demonstrated (Fig. 1) the appearance of a fast migrating material in the plasmin treated C5 which was only present in quite small amounts

71

in the control. This small amount of fast migrating material was also found in C5 which had not previously been incubated at 37°C. Hemolytic titration demonstrated (Fig. 1) that the conversion of C5 into electrophoretically fast material coincided with a 70 per cent reduction of its hemolytic activity.

In subsequent studies, this experiment was repeated using a buffer of a pH of 8·5 (veronal). In this case, complete conversion of C5 into an immunoelectrophoretically fast component was observed. If this same reaction was performed in the presence of added epsilon amino caproic acid (EACA) at 0·3 M concentration, conversion of C5 was prevented entirely.

Isolation of C5. Since plasmin had been shown to affect C5, and since plg/pln was demonstrated in C5 preparations isolated according to Nilsson and Müller-Eberhard (1965), special efforts were made to find conditions for a more efficient separation of plg/pln from C5. Advantage was therefore taken of the capacity of *l*-lysine and epsilon amino caproic acid (EACA) to increase the solubility of plg/pln, to prevent activation of plg, as well as to improve the chromatographic separation of plg/pln from other serum proteins (Mosesson, 1962; Alkjaersig *et al.*, 1959).

Table 1 summarizes the new, three step procedure for the isolation of C5 from human serum. Details of the procedure are given in the Materials and Methods section.

The euglobulin fraction obtained in the first step of the new purification procedure constitutes between 1–1·5% of the total protein and contains (determined by the Folin procedure) approximately 35% of the C5 and only 0·5% of the plg/pln (determined by radial diffusion) present in the starting serum. The corresponding figures for the euglobulin fraction obtained by the old procedure (Nilsson and Müller-Eberhard, 1965) were 3–3·5, 40 and 50% respectively. The time allowed for the precipitation in the new procedure was determined in preliminary studies, which indicated maximal yields of C5 and minimal co-precipitation of plg/pln after 3·5 hr.

The euglobulin was separated by TEAE cellulose chromatography into four main fractions (Table 1, step No. 2 and Fig. 2). The first of these is represented by the relatively low protein peak in test tube No. 1 through 70 which coincides

Table 1. Purification of human C5

1. Preparation of euglobulin	*Dilution:* Serum (1 vol), 0·11 M *l*-lysine (2·7 vol) and water (approx. 1·45 vol) to bring conductance to 4·1 at 4°C
	Acidification: 1 M acetic acid to bring pH to 5·0.
	Precipitation: Stirring at 4°C for 3·5 hr
2. TEAE cellulose chromatography	NaCl gradient elution at constant pH of 7·0 in 0·03 M PO_4 and 0·1 M EACA. Conductance 2·5–9·0 mMho at 4°C.
3. OH apatite chromatography	PO_4 gradient elution at constant pH of 7·9 in 0·1 M EACA. Conductance 3·0–15·5 at 4°C.

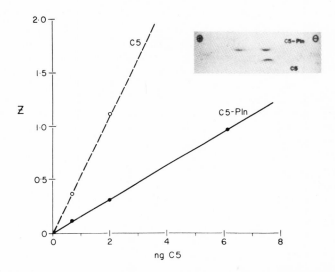

Fig. 1. Plasmin induced modification of human C5. $50\,\mu g$ of human C5 were incubated at 37°C for 1 hr in 0·1 ml veronal buffered saline, pH 7·4, in the presence or in the absence (= control) of $5\,\mu g$ human plasmin. The plasmin treated material (C5-pln) retained only 30 per cent of the activity of the control (C5), when tested hemolytically (conversion of 3×10^7 EACl4^{oxy}23 to EACl4^{oxy}235, lyseable upon addition of C6–C9, expressed as the average no. of hits, Z). Immunoelectrophoresis using a monospecific anti C5 antiserum, demonstrated the appearance of an electrophoretically fast conversion product in the plasmin treated material (C5-pln) not seen in the control (C5).

with the fall through fraction of the eluate. This peak is followed in sequence by a distinct protein peak in test tubes No. 126–170, by a less conspicuous peak in test tubes No. 180–240, and finally by the dominant peak of the eluate in tubes No. 250 through the end. Hemolytic tests (not shown on Fig. 2) showed the presence of C5 in the second peak (tubes No. 126–170). Double diffusion tests demonstrated a similar distribution of C5 but also the presence of C3 and $\beta 1H$ in the same fractions. Ten to fifteen per cent of the eluted protein was recovered in tube fractions No. 126–170. Plg/pln was eluted mainly in the first peak of the eluate but due to trailing it also contaminated later fractions throughout the eluate of the column. Despite this incomplete separation, the described chromatographic procedure was relatively efficient in removing plg/pln from C5. The same degree of separation of these factors could not be accomplished when EACA was deleted from the eluting buffer. In this case, plg/pln was retained longer on the column and had a relatively greater tendency of trailing. Since the chromatographic property of other proteins appeared to be unaffected this resulted in considerable overlap between the latter part of the peak of maximal fibrinolytic activity and the leading part of the C5 peak.

The C5-containing fractions (No. 126–170) of the eluate of the TEAE cellulose column were pooled and further separated by OH apatite chromatography (Step No. 3, Table 1 and Fig. 3). This pool contained some 0·07% of the total protein of the original starting serum. Protein analysis of the eluate from the OH

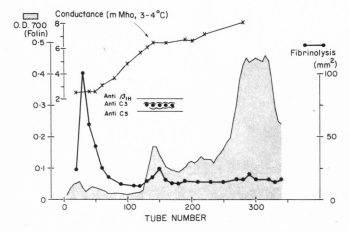

Fig. 2. Purification of C5. Separation of euglobulin of a prefraction of C5 (see text) by TEAE cellulose chromatography. Column: $4·35 \times 35$ cm. Linear gradient elution: 2·5l. of starting buffer consisting of PO_4 at pH 7·0, 0·03 M, containing 0·1 M EACA, conductance 2·5 mMho at 4°C and 2·5 l. limiting buffer with NaCl added to adjust conductance to 9·0 mMho at 4°C. C5 demonstrable by double diffusion (graphically recorded) was found in mixture with C3 and $\beta 1H$ corresponding to a distinct protein peak (test tubes 126–170) and was well separated from the early peak containing the bulk of plasminogen (demonstrated fibrinolytically) and the two later peaks containing the bulk of the protein of the separated euglobulin.

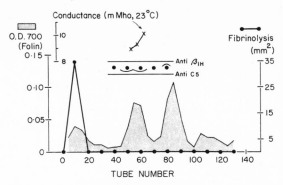

Fig. 3. Purification of C5. Isolation by OH apatite chromatography of a prefraction of C5 obtained from TEAE cellulose chromatography (a portion of the pool of test tube fraction 126 through 170, Fig. 2). Column width = 2 cm, volume (ml) = $1 \cdot 2 \times$ No. of mg applied protein. Linear gradient elution: starting buffer consisting of sodium potassium PO_4 at pH $7 \cdot 9$ and conductance of 3 mMho at 4°C (5 mMho at 23°C) containing $0 \cdot 1\,M$ EACA and limiting buffer consisting of a similar PO_4 buffer at a conductance of $15 \cdot 5$ mMho at 4°C (25 mMho at 23°C). C5, demonstrable by double diffusion tests (graphically recorded) was obtained in a distinct protein peak (test tubes 50–62) well separated from other proteins of the eluate.

apatite showed four well-separated protein peaks. The first one of these (test tubes No. 1–20) was relatively small and was found to contain all of the demonstrable fibrinolytic activity of the eluate. The second, relatively large protein peak (test tubes No. 45–65) contained C5, demonstrable immunochemically and hemolytically and constituted approximately 30% of the protein eluted from that column. The third and major peak (test tubes No. 75–95) of the eluate contained $\beta1H$, and the fourth (test tubes No. 100–125), relatively small protein peak contained C3. A complete separation of C5 from C3, $\beta1H$ and the residual plg/pln contamination was therefore accomplished in this final step of purification. This fractionation step was also enhanced by the presence of EACA. When EACA was present the plg/pln was eluted before C5. When EACA was not present the plg/pln was eluted with and partially after C5. The yield of purified C5 by the new preparation method varied from 1 to 2 mg per 100 ml processed serum.

Characterization by immunochemical and fibrinolytic assay procedures of C5 isolated by the new purification method. Immunochemical homogeneity of purified C5 was tested by the Ouchterlony technique and by immune electrophoresis. Undiluted (0·6 mg/ml) of C5 and two-fold dilutions thereof were reacted with undiluted and two-fold dilutions of potent antisera against human serum proteins (Fig. 4). A strong precipitine band formed with the anti-C5 and a weak band with anti-whole serum, but no bands were discernable with anti-C3, anti-$\beta1H$, anti IgG, anti IgA or anti IgM. The band developing with anti whole serum was identified as a C5 anti-C5 precipitin line. Immunoelectrophoretic analysis of the purified C5 against anti-C5 disclosed a symmetric precipitin arc in the β region. Using these criteria, immunochemical homogeneity of the purified C5 was established.

The fibrinolytic assay failed to demonstrate plg/pln in the purified C5 isolated

Ouchterlony Analysis of Purified Human C5

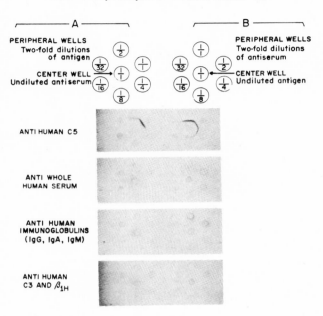

Fig. 4. Analysis of purified C5. Test for antigenic homogeneity by the double diffusion technique. Undiluted antisera were reacted with 2-fold serial dilutions of antigen (purified C5, undiluted 0·6 mg/ml) (A), or undiluted antigen was reacted with 2-fold serial dilutions of the antisera (B). Only with anti human C5 antiserum was a strong precipitin band demonstrable. The weak precipitin band developed with anti whole human serum was caused by antibodies to C5 present in relatively low titers in this antiserum.

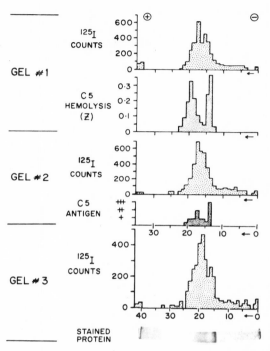

Fig. 5. Analysis of purified C5. Properties when separated by polyacrylamide gel (5%) electrophoresis in the absence of SDS. 30 μg of C5 (6% ^{125}I-labelled and 94% non-labelled) were separated simultaneously in three different gels. C5, as measured by staining (gel # 3), by hemolytic activity (gel # 1) or by the double diffusion technique (gel # 2) was found to distribute in a similar, bimodal fashion, in a relatively fast diffuse and a relatively slow, sharp zone. The radioactivity was found mainly in segments corresponding to the faster one of these zones. Direction of migration indicated by arrow.

77

Polyacrylamide Gel Electrophoresis of Human C5 in the presence of Sodium Dodecyl Sulfate

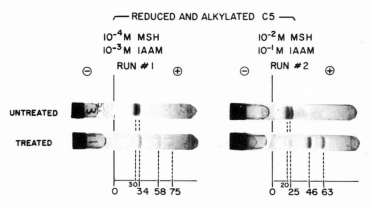

Fig. 6. Analysis of purified C5: Properties when separated by polyacrylamide gel (7·5%) electrophoresis in the presence of SDS. Non-reduced material (runs # 1 and # 2, untreated) migrated as two relatively slow bands (the 'paired bands'). Modification of the electrophoretic properties followed reduction with mercaptoethanol (MSH) and subsequent alkylation with iodoacetamide (IAAM) in 10x molar excess. MSH at 10^{-4} M concentration (run # 1) converted the material, mainly into a single band, corresponding to the fast member of the 'paired bands'. MSH at 10^{-2} M concentration (run # 2) converted the material into two well-separated bands, of faster migration than any band seen in the non-reduced preparations. Direction of migration towards the right.

by the new technique. The maximal level of plg/pln contamination was therefore below 1/10,000 w/w).

Characterization of C5 by polyacrylamide gel electrophoresis. The results of a poly-acrylamide gel electrophoretic analysis (according to Davis, 1964) (See Methods, condition (a)) of isolated C5 are recorded in Fig. 5. To each of three polyacrylamide gels, approximately $2\,\mu g$ ^{125}I-labelled and $30\,\mu g$ non-labelled C5 were applied. After electrophoresis, one of the gels was stained. A characteristic pattern of a sharp, slowly migrating stained band (approx. segment 15, gel No. 3, Fig. 5) and a faster migrating, wide and more diffuse, stained zone were seen (approx. segment 17–25, gel No. 3, Fig. 5). Cut segments of the stained gel were counted, and the counts were recorded on a scale corresponding to the photographic image of the stained gel. The radioactivity and the protein stain were found in approximately the same area of the gel, however, with the maximum of the radioactivity tending to correspond to the faster migrating portion of the stained pattern. Gels No. 1 and 2 were also cut into segments, but without previous staining. Their radioactivity showed the same distribution as that of the stained gels, indicating similar electrophoretic migration in all three gels.

Eluates from segments of the non-stained gels were analyzed for C5 hemolytically (gel No. 1) and immunochemically (gel No. 2). Both assays indicated a bimodal distribution of C5 corresponding to that indicated by the protein stain of gel No. 3. Polyacrylamide gel electrophoresis analysis of C5 in the absence of SDS gave identical results with C5 isolated by both the old and new methods.

The following conclusions were drawn from this experiment: (a) Since no antigen other than the C5 antigen was demonstrable in the analyzed preparation, and since this antigen was demonstrable in all areas of the gels which could be stained for proteins, the heterogeneity was not due to any extraneous protein contaminate, but rather due to a heterogeneity of C5; (b) Since C5 hemolytic activity was demonstrable in all areas of the gels containing C5, the observed heterogeneity was not caused by degradation leading to physical and functional modification of the protein; (c) The trace of C5 which was ^{125}I-labelled behaved differently than the bulk of C5, detected by the staining, the double diffusion or by the hemolytic assay procedures.

Considerable reduction of this apparent physical heterogeneity was observed when the polyacrylamide gel electrophoretic analysis of isolated C5 was performed in the presence of SDS (see Methods, condition (b)) and Fig. 6). The top two gels depicted in this figures ('untreated') represent two different experiments. Instead of the broad, diffuse, stained pattern shown in Fig. 5, each gel now showed a distinct pattern of only a pair of bands at close distance to each other. The bands, the 'paired bands' had migrated 30–34 per cent and 20–25 per cent of the length of the gels of the two separate runs. Therefore although there was a considerable reduction of the apparent heterogeneity of C5 in the presence of SDS, still some electrophoretic heterogeneity remained in the presence of SDS.

If the same electrophoretic analysis was performed after reduction and alkylation (see Methods) of C5, this protein pattern was modified (see the lower, 'treated' gels of Fig. 6). After reduction of C5 at a MSH concentration of $10^{-4}\,M$, the cathodal member of the 'paired bands' disappeared whereas the anodal member (the faster) of the bands remained often as the only protein band detectable in the gel. Sometimes however trace amounts of the two more rapidly migrating bands were also observed (Fig. 6, lower gel, run No. 1) (c.f., below).

After reduction at a higher MSH concentration ($10^{-2}\,M$) both of the two 'paired bands' almost totally disappeared. Instead, two-well separated more rapidly migrating bands appeared (Fig. 6, lower gel, run No. 2). A pattern of these two faster bands was also observed when C5 was reduced at a higher concentration of MSH ($0 \cdot 14\,M$) in a solution containing 1% SDS and subsequently separated by polyacrylamide gel electrophoresis in the presence of excess MSH and $0 \cdot 1$% SDS, as described by Weber and Osborn (1969). This finding therefore indicated that the observed, electrophoretically faster migrating bands constituted the subunit polypeptides of the C5 molecule. In order to determine the molecular weight of these subunits three independent molecular weight determinations were performed according to Weber and Osborn (1969) (Fig. 7). The following markers of known polypeptide molecular weight, were used: Myosin (220000), Phosphorylase-a (94000), Human Serum Albumin (68000), IgG H chain (50000) (Weber and Osborn, 1969). In graphs plotting relative migration (abcissa) vs. log molecular weight (ordinate) a straight line connected the polypeptide molecular weights of the IgG H-chain, the albumin and the phosphorylase-a markers. The point for myosin fell above the extension of this line in the higher molecular weight range. By visual fitting a hyperbolic standard curve was constructed. On the basis of this curve the mean molecular weight of the fast

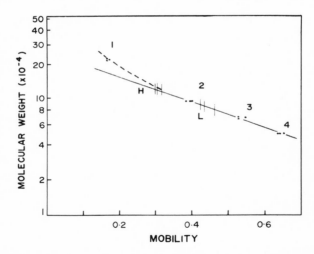

Fig. 7. Determination of the molecular weights of the polypeptide chains of human C5. The results of three independent polyacrylamide gel electrophoretic runs are recorded. The standard curve was constructed by connecting the points for the markers of known polypeptide molecular weights: (1) Myosin, (2) Phosphorylase-a, (3) Serum Albumin and (4) IgG H-chain. 'H' and 'L' denotes the intercepts between the standard curve and the electrophoretic migration of the C5 H- and L-chains respectively. Abscissa: Relative distance of electrophoresis migration. Ordinate: Molecular weight.

migrating C5 subunit (L-chain) was determined to be 83000 (80–87000) and that of the slowly migrating C5 subunit (H-chain 123000 (120–125000) (Fig. 7).

Gel filtration of non-reduced and of reduced and alkylated C5 in the presence of SDS. A mixture of ^{125}I-labelled (6%) and non-labelled (94%) non-reduced purified C5, as well as C5 which had been reduced ($10^{-2}\,M$ MSH) and alkylated was treated with SDS and analyzed in separate experiments by Sepharose 6B gel filtrations (see Materials and Methods). Both the non-reduced as well as the reduced and alkylated materials were eluted in single, bell-shaped peaks from the column. The K_{av} of non-reduced C5 was found to be 0·21 and that of reduced and alkylated C5 was 0·27. This change of K_{av} corresponded to a decrease of the molecular weight of the reduced and alkylated material by approximately 50 per cent. Non-reduced C5 which had previously been separated by Sepharose 6B gel filtration was further analyzed by polyacrylamide gel electrophoresis in the presence of SDS. Concentrated fractions obtained from the early and late halves of the eluted single peak gave the same protein pattern (the 'paired bands', c.f. Fig. 6) characteristic for non-reduced C5, which had not previously exposed to Sepharose 6B gel filtration. Similar electrophoretic analysis was performed on the Sepharose 6B separated reduced ($10^{-2}\,M$ MSH) and alkylated C5. The early and the late half of the eluted peak contained both of the two fast migrating bands demonstrable by the electrophoretic analysis of reduced ($10^{-2}\,M$ MSH) and alkylated C5 (c.f. Fig. 6, run No. 2 lower gel). However, the early half of the peak contained a relatively higher concentration of the electrophoretically *slow* band whereas the late half of the peak contained a relatively higher concentration of the *fast* band.

DISCUSSION

This paper describes a modified procedure for the isolation of human C5 in quantities adequate for chemical studies. It also records some studies on the physical nature of C5 determined by analytical polyacrylamide gel electrophoresis.

By modifying the procedure employed in the previously described isolation technique (Nilsson and Müller-Eberhard, 1965) a considerably improved method was elaborated. Both procedures start with the precipitation of a euglobulin fraction from whole serum. In the new procedure this was done in the presence of *l*-lysine under conditions (pH and ionic strength) which otherwise corresponded to those described by Nelson and coworkers (1966) for the precipitation of guinea pig C5. The fraction obtained contained approximately 35 per cent of the C5 and only 1·5% of the total protein of the starting serum. Two distinct advantages of this new euglobulin preparation were observed: (1) The amount of contaminating proteins were reduced to allow a simplification of the subsequent preparative procedures. Only two subsequent chromatographic steps are necessary for completion (see Table 1), whereas the old method required an additional step of preparative electrophoresis, (2) The presence of *l*-lysine during precipitation specifically reduced the amounts of coprecipitated plasminogen/ plasmin (plg/pln). Approximately half of the serum plg/pln was precipitated as a euglobulin by the old method, whereas only 0·5% was precipitated by the new method. The effects of *l*-lysine and of EACA are the same. Both substances have the ability to specifically increase the solubility of plg/pln, prevent the aggregation of plg/pln with other proteins, and prevent activation of plasminogen to plasmin (Mosesson, 1962, Alkjaersig *et al.*, 1959). By presumably limiting the tendency of plg/pln to form aggregates with other proteins, a more distinct chromatographic behavior, favorable for the separation, was also achieved (see Figs. 2 and 3). The presence of *l*-lysine or EACA in buffers utilized during the preparation also protected against activation of plasminogen and subsequent degradation of C5. The latter consideration is probably an important one, since it was shown that plasmin indeed degraded C5 into a hemolytically inactive product (see Fig. 1). Preparations of C5 purified under these new conditions contained no plg/pln detectable by the fibrinolytic assay. The tests were performed at a protein concentration range of 1–2 mg/ml, which excluded contamination with plg/pln at levels exceeding 1 : 10,000 (w/w).

C5 preparations obtained by the new method appeared homogeneous when analyzed by immune electrophoresis and by the double diffusion technique (see Fig. 4). Despite this immunochemical evidence for homogeneity, physical heterogeneity was suggested in analyses by polyacrylamide gel electrophoresis (in the absence of SDS) (see Fig. 5). The fact that stained protein, C5 antigen, as well as C5 hemolytic activity were equally distributed in these gels suggested that aggregation of active C5 rather than degradation and inactivation of C5 was the most plausible cause of the apparent heterogeneity. This interpretation was supported by the previous observation that C5 undergoes concentration dependent, reversible aggregation upon analytical ultracentrifugation (Nilsson and Müller-Eberhard, 1965) as well as upon Sephadex G 200 gel filtration (Nilsson, unpublished observation). Dissociating agents were therefore expected to eliminate this heterogeneity by resolving the aggregates. This effect was indeed observed in that purified C5 behaved as a single molecular species when subjected to Sepharose 6B gel filtration in the presence of SDS.

Despite this evidence for homogeneity in molecular size, polyacrylamide gel electrophoresis performed on non-reduced C5 in the presence of SDS, indicated some residual heterogeneity in that a pair of bands, rather than a single band were observed (see Fig. 6). This heterogeneity, however, could not be associated with molecular size heterogeneity; for non-reduced C5 recovered from any portion of the eluate of the Sepharose 6B column (containing SDS) displayed identical 'paired band' patterns upon SDS-polyacrylamide gel electrophoresis. Therefore, the question was raised whether a heterogeneity in charge could explain this electrophoretic pattern. Under the conditions employed in these experiments, the electric charge was strongly dependent on the amount of SDS that could bind to the protein. One known factor influencing the binding of SDS to a given protein is to what degree its disulfide bonds are reduced. Reduction of disulfide bonds has been shown invariably to lead to an increased SDS binding and consequently greater electronegative charge by allowing access of the detergent to otherwise covered portions of the molecule (Pitt-Rivers and Impiombato, 1968). In the case of C5 the conversion of the slower into the electrophoretically faster of the 'paired bands' following mild reduction ($10^{-4} M$ MSH) (Fig. 6, run No. 1) indeed suggested that this treatment lead to an increase of the negative *charge* of the protein, since the 'paired bands' pattern could not be associated with molecular *size* heterogeneity. Our tentative interpretation is that this was caused by the dissociation of a labile disulfide bond or by a structural change due to disulfide interchange allowing more SDS to bind to the C5 protein. Since the electrophoretically fast component is present in preparations not previously exposed to MSH, this change appears to occur spontaneously.

We conclude from these studies that the apparent heterogeneity of the isolated C5 observed in analysis performed *in the absence* of SDS can be accounted for by reversible aggregation and that the heterogeneity seen in the *presence of SDS* may be accounted for by partial spontaneous reduction of the protein or perhaps by a disulfide interchain reaction not associated with change of the molecular size of the protein. From these studies we also conclude that the purity and characteristics of this C5 preparation has been defined, and it can now be employed in further studies of the physical chemical and functional properties of human C5.

Finally, it should be noted that new information concerning the subunit structure of C5 was obtained in the present study. Reduction with MSH under conditions shown to efficiently degrade proteins into their polypeptide subunits (Weber and Osborn, 1969) was found to yield two C5 subunits. The molecular weights of these subunits determined according to Weber and Osborn (1969) were 83000 (80–87000) and 123000 (120–125000) respectively. Since native human C5 was eluted from Sephadex G-200 columns in fractions corresponding to a molecular weight of approximately 200000 (Nilsson, unpublished observation) and since Sepharose 6B gel filtration in the presence of SDS indicated that treatment of C5 with MSH (10^{-2} M) and iodoacetamide (see Fig. 6, run No. 2) was associated with a reduction of the molecular weight by approximately 50%, it appears that the C5 molecule is composed of one of each of the above chains. Consequently the C5 molecular weight is approximately 206000.

Acknowledgements — This work was supported by grants AM 13515 NIH, HE 10-907 NIH, and the John Hartford Foundation. The authors wish to thank Mary Batt, Julia Mapes and Randy Nelson for their excellent technical assistance.

REFERENCES

Alkjaersig N., Fletcher A. P. and Sherry S. (1959) *J. biol. Chem.* **234**, 832.

Cook C. T., Shin H. S., Mayer M. M. and Laundenslayer K. A. (1971) *J. Immun.* **106**, 467.

Cooper N. R. and Müller-Eberhard H. J. (1970) *J. exp. Med.* **132**, 775.

Davis B. J. (1964) *Ann. N.Y. Acad. Sci.* **121**, 404.

Hayward B. J. and Augustin R. (1957) *Int. Archs Allergy appl. Immun.* **11**, 192.

Kunkel H. G. and Tiselius A. (1951) *J. gen. Physiol.* **35**, 89.

Mancini G., Vaerman J. P., Carbonara A. O. and Heremans J. F. (1964) *Protides of the Biological Fluids*, Proceedings of the 11th Colloquium, Bruges, 1963 (Edited by Peeters H.), p. 370. Elsevier, Amsterdam.

Mayer M. M. (1961) *Experimental Immunochemistry* (Edited by Kabat E. A. and Mayer M. M.), p. 133. Thomas, Springfield, Ill.

McConahey P. J. and Dixon F. J. (1966) *Int. Archs Allergy* **29**, 185.

Mosesson M. W. (1962) *Biochim. biophys. Acta* **57**, 204.

Nelson R. A., Jensen J., Gigli J. and Tamura N. (1966) *Immunochemistry* **3**, 111.

Nilsson U. R. and Müller-Eberhard H. J. (1965) *J. exp. Med.* **122**, 277.

Nilsson U. R. and Müller-Eberhard H. J. (1967) *J. exp. Med.* **125**, 1.

Nilsson U. R. and Miller M. E. (1971) *J. clin. Invest.* (manuscript submitted).

Pitt-Rivers R. and Impiombato F. S. A. (1968) *Biochem. J.* **109**, 825.
Scheidegger J. J. (1955) *Int. Archs Allergy appl. Immun.* **33**, 11.
Stroud R. M. (1971) *J. Lab. clin. Med.* **77**, 645.
Tiselius A., Hjerten S. and Levin O. (1956) *Archs Biochem. Biophys.* **65**, 132.
Tomar R. and Taylor F. B., Jr. (1971) *J. biol. Chem.* (in press).
Weber K. and Osborn M. (1969) *J. biol. Chem.* **244**, 4406.

ISOLATION OF THE SIXTH COMPONENT OF COMPLEMENT FROM HUMAN SERUM*†

CARLOS M. ARROYAVE and HANS J. MÜLLER-EBERHARD

Abstract— Using DEAE and hydroxyapatite chromatography and Pevikon block electrophoresis the sixth component of complement (C6) was isolated from human serum. The protein was shown to be homogeneous on disc and immunoelectrophoresis. It constitutes a β_2-globulin with a molecular weight of 95,000. Dose response experiments showed proportionality between $a - \ln(1-y)$ and input of isolated C6. The number of molecules per cell required to achieve $a - \ln(1-y)$ value of unity was inversely proportional to the number of C4, 2, 3, 5-sites present on the assay cells. The final isolation product, although resembling physically and immunologically C6 in fresh serum, was less active than the latter. The possibility exists that a cofactor which enhances C6 hemolytic activity was removed during purification. Employing the described procedure, C6 was also isolated from rabbit and guinea pig serum.

INTRODUCTION

Methods of isolation have been reported for all human complement proteins except for C6 and C7. The purpose of this paper is to describe a procedure which allows purification of C6 from human, rabbit and guinea pig serum as a physicochemically and immunochemically homogeneous protein. The C6 protein is of particular biochemical and biological interest: It has the capacity to form functionally relevant complexes with C5 and C7 (Nilsson and Müller-Eberhard, 1967). It is a subunit of the high molecular weight chemotactic factor for polymorphonuclear leukocytes (Ward et al., 1966; Lachmann et al., 1970). It is absent from the plasma of a strain of rabbits with an inherited complement deficiency (Rother et al., 1966; Nelson and Biro, 1968; Lachmann, 1970). It participates in the mechanism of normal blood coagulation (Zimmerman et al., 1971) and it is required for the initiation and acceleration of blood coagulation by immune complexes and cell wall products of gram negative bacteria (Zimmerman and Müller-Eberhard 1971). In fact, recognition of some of its biological functions was possible only after isolation of the protein in this laboratory. Part of the material to be presented was published in the form of an abstract (Arroyave and Müller-Eberhard, 1970).

MATERIALS AND METHODS

Serum and purified complement components. Serum was obtained from two units

*This is publication number 501 from the Department of Experimental Pathology, Scripps Clinic and Research Foundation, La Jolla, Calif. 92037, U.S.A.

†This work was supported by United States Public Health Service Grant Al-07007, United States Atomic Energy Commission Contract AT(04-3)-730 and American Heart Association, Inc. Grant 68-666.

of human blood. After coagulation the clot was removed by centrifugation, leaving approximately 400 ml of serum. The pH was adjusted to 7·0 and the conductance to 3·0 mmho/cm with 1 N HCl and cold distilled water. This material was kept at 4° for 1 hr, and the resulting precipitate (euglobulin) was removed by centrifugation at 1200 **g** and 4° for 1 hr. The precipitate was used to obtain macromolecular C1 (Nelson et al., 1966) and the supernate (pseudoglobulin) to isolate C6.

C2 (Polley and Müller-Eberhard, 1968), C3 (Nilsson and Müller-Eberhard, 1965), C4 (Müller-Eberhard and Biro, 1963), C5 (Nilsson and Müller-Eberhard, 1965), C7 (Götze and Müller-Eberhard, 1970), C8 (Manni and Müller-Eberhard, 1969) and C9 (Hadding and Müller-Eberhard, 1969) were isolated using methodology described in the indicated references.

Diluent. Isotonic veronal buffered saline containing Ca^{++} and Mg^{++}(VB), pH 7·4, was used as such or supplemented with 0·1 per cent (w/v) gelatin (VBG) (Kabat and Mayer, 1961).

Hemolytic assay of C6

1. *Assay with C6 deficient rabbit serum.* (Rother et al., 1966). 10–50 μl of sample, C6 deficient rabbit serum in a final dilution of 1/40 with VBG, 100 μl of VBG and 100 μl of EA (5×10^8 sensitized sheep erythrocytes/ml) were mixed and incubated at 37° for 30 min. The reaction was stopped by the addition of 1·5 ml cold saline and by immediate centrifugation. Free hemoglobin was quantitated spectrophotometrically at 412 nm or 541 nm.

2. *Assay with purified complement components.* EACl,4, ^{oxy}2,3 was prepared as described (Nilsson and Müller-Eberhard, 1965). 0·2 ml of this cell suspension ($1·5 \times 10^8$ cells/ml) was mixed with 2 μg of C5, 4 μg of C7 and varying amounts of test material. The mixture was incubated for 20 min at 37°, centrifuged, and the cells were washed twice with cold VBG. The cells were then incubated for 60 min at 37° in 0·4 ml VBG containing an excess of C8 and C9. The degree of hemolysis was quantitated as above.

Labeling of C6 with radioactive iodine. C6 was labeled with ^{125}I by the method of McConahey and Dixon (1966). The specific radioactivity was approximately 10,000 cpm/μg and the loss of hemolytic activity did not exceed 20 per cent.

Preparation of monospecific antiserum to C6. Rabbits were immunized by injection of 100 μl of a mixture containing equal volumes of purified human C6 (20 μg) and complete Freund's adjuvant into a popliteal lymph node (Goudie et al., 1966). One month later, 200 μl of a similar mixture with 100 μg of C6 was injected intramuscularly and subcutaneously, and 8 days after the animals were bled. Rabbit anti-rabbit C6 was produced by the same method using purified rabbit C6 and C6 deficient rabbits.

C6 protein determination. Protein was quantitated by the Folin method (Folin and Ciocalteu, 1927); C3 was used arbitrarily as the standard.

Immunochemical analysis. Immunologic analysis of C6 preparations was performed in Ouchterlony plates (Ouchterlony, 1967) using antisera against γG-, γA-, γM-globulin, transferrin, albumin and whole human serum which were purchased from Behringwerke AG, Marburg/Lahn, Germany. Monospecific antisera to C3, C4, C5 and C8 (Nilsson and Müller-Eberhard, 1965; Müller-

Eberhard and Biro, 1963; Manni and Müller-Eberhard, 1969) were prepared as described. Immunoelectrophoresis was performed according to Scheidegger (1955) using either 2 per cent agar or agarose. Immunochemical quantitation of C6 was performed using the single radial diffusion technique of Mancini *et al.* (1965).

Polyacrylamide gel electrophoresis. For disc electrophoresis on polyacrylamide gels, the method of Davis (1964) was used employing a polyacrylamide concentration of 6 per cent in the separation gel. To locate C6 hemolytic activity after disc electrophoresis, the gel was sliced longitudinally, one half was stained for protein, the other was cut into 2 mm segments, each of which was transferred to a 1 × 7 cm tube containing 0·5 ml of VBG. After 12 hr at 4°, the eluates were analyzed for C6 hemolytic activity.

Molecular weight determination. The molecular weight of C6 was estimated by:
1. The polyacrylamide gel electrophoresis method of Hedrick and Smith (1968) using a gel concentration range of 4–12 per cent, and bromphenol blue as a marker of the buffer front. As reference proteins with known molecular weight were used the monomer, dimer and trimer of human serum albumin (Behringwerke AG, Marburg/Lahn, Germany).

2. The diffusion coefficient (D) was estimated according to Andrews (1965) using a 3 × 100 cm Sephadex G-200 column equilibrated with VB. The sedimentation coefficient (s) was determined by sucrose density ultracentrifugation according to Kunkel (1960) employing a 7–31 per cent linear sucrose gradient and phosphate buffer, pH 7·0, ionic strength 0·15. Human thyroglobulin, C8, γG and hemoglobin were used as reference substances. The molecular weight was calculated from s and D assuming a partial specific volume of 0·73.

Determination of the C6 dose response. EACl-3 cells were prepared which contained 3000 $C\overline{4,2}$ molecular complexes per cell. Tubes containing various dilutions of the purified C6 were charged with 1 μg C5, 10 μg C7 and 3 × 10^7 EACl-3 cells. The final volume was 500 μl and the tubes were incubated for 20 min at 37°. After incubation the tubes were centrifuged and the cells washed twice with cold VBG. Then, C8 (6 ng) and C9 (10 ng) were added and the tubes incubated at 37° for 60 min. Following the second incubation, 1 ml of cold isotonic saline solution was added to each tube, the tubes were centrifuged and the A 541 of the supernate was determined. The degree of hemolysis, y, was converted to the average number of sites per cell, z, according to Mayer (Kabat and Mayer, 1961).

Isolation procedure. The pseudoglobulin of 400 ml serum was applied to a 5 × 100 cm column of packed DEAE-cellulose, equilibrated with phosphate buffer, pH 7·0, having a conductance of 3·0 mmho/cm (starting buffer). The adsorbed protein was eluted with a NaCl concentration gradient (2 l. of starting buffer and 2 l. of the same buffer adjusted to 30 mmho/cm with NaCl). The flow rate was 120 ml/hr and 15 ml fractions were collected. The fractions containing C6 activity were pooled and dialyzed against the starting buffer in order to be rechromatographed on a 2·5 × 50 cm DEAE-cellulose column. The protein was eluted with a linear gradient prepared with 1 liter of starting buffer and 1 liter of the same buffer containing NaCl that yielded a conductance of 20 mmho/cm.

The material containing C6 activity was concentrated and divided into two aliquots, each of which was subjected to preparative electrophoresis on a $18 \times 36 \times 1 \cdot 5$ cm Pevikon block, using barbital buffer, pH 8·6, $T/2 = 0·05$ (Müller–Eberhard, 1960). Electrophoresis was performed at 4° for 36 hr at a potential gradient of 4 v/cm. The block was cut into 1·25 cm segments and eluted with phosphate buffer, pH 7·9, 8·0 mmho/cm. The eluates with C6 activity were pooled, concentrated to 20 ml and applied to a $1 \cdot 6 \times 30$ cm hydroxyapatite column. The hydroxyapatite was made according to Tiselius *et al.* (1956), and chromatography was performed according to the procedure described previously (Nilsson and Müller-Eberhard, 1965). A stepwise elution chromatography was performed with sodium phosphate buffers of constant pH (7·9) and increasing conductance (8, 10, 11, 11·25 mmho/cm).

Since at this stage the protein concentration in the column effluent was low, siliconized tubes were used for collection of the fractions. The C6 pool was passed through a Millipore filter ($0 \cdot 45\,\mu$) and then concentrated, and the final product was stored in the elution buffer or in VB without Ca^{++} and Mg^{++} after quick freezing in liquid nitrogen.

To concentrate protein solutions, an Amicon pressure filtration device and a UM 50 membrane (Amicon Corp., Lexington, Mass.) were used To prevent bacterial growth during the isolation procedure which usually lasted 20 days, all the buffers used for chromatography and electrophoresis contained $5 \times 10^{-2}\,M$ chloramphenicol (Parke, Davis and Co., Ann Arbor, Mich.) and $2 \cdot 5 \times 10^{-5}\,M$ Kanamycin sulfate (Bristol Laboratories, Syracuse, N.Y.).

RESULTS

Isolation. Preliminary experiments revealed that removal of the euglobulin from human serum at pH 7·0 or 8·0 left at least 90 per cent of the C6 hemolytic activity in the supernate pseudoglobulin fraction (Table 1). These experiments also showed a marked variation in the stability of C6 activity at different pH values. Samples of whole human serum, or in later experiments purified C6, were exposed at 4° to various hydrogen ion concentrations for periods up to 24 hr. Aliquots were withdrawn at certain time intervals, the pH of the samples was adjusted to 7·5 and residual C6 activity was assayed immediately. As shown in Fig. 1, C6 activity was rapidly destroyed at pH 5 and 6, but was virtually stable

Table 1. Distribution of C6 hemolytic activity in euglobulin and pseudo-globulin produced under different conditions

Solvent	pH	Distribution of C6 activity	
		Euglobulin (%)	Pseudoglobulin (%)
0·01 M acetate buffer	5·0	50–60	40–50
0·008 M EDTA solution	5·4	50	50
0·01 M phosphate buffer	6·0	25–30	70–75
0·01 M phosphate buffer	7·0	8–10	90–92
0·01 M phosphate buffer	8·0	5–10	90–95

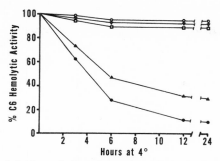

Fig. 1. Stability of the hemolytic activity of purified C6 or of C6 contained in whole human serum as a function of exposure to various hydrogen ion concentrations (pH 5 ●, 6 ▲, 7 □, 8 ○ and 9 ▽).

at pH 7, 8 or 9. Therefore, the isolation procedure was designed so that all operations could be performed in buffers of pH 7·0–8·6.

Following euglobulin precipitation at pH 7·0, the pseudoglobulin was applied to a DEAE-cellulose column. The adsorbed protein was eluted with a NaCl gradient (Fig. 2). The fractions representing the peak of C6 activity were pooled and chromatographed on a second DEAE column under similar conditions (Fig. 3).

The concentrated pool of C6 from the second DEAE column was then subjected to preparative electrophoresis on a Pevikon block (Fig. 4). C6 activity was eluted from the β-globulin region, and the eluates corresponding to the peak of the C6 activity were pooled and applied to a hydroxyapatite column (Fig. 5). During stepwise elution, C6 activity corresponding to a discrete protein peak appeared in the final step. This material was concentrated, divided into small aliquots and stored at −70° for future analysis. The same procedure could be employed for the isolation of C6 from rabbit and guinea pig serum.

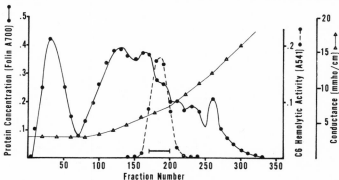

Fig. 2. First chromatographic procedure of C6 isolation using DEAE-cellulose. Column size, 5 × 100 cm; starting buffer, phosphate, pH 7·0, 3·0 mmho/cm. Elution of pseudoglobulins was accomplished with a NaCl gradient from 3·0–30·0 mmho/cm. Fractions 170–200 which contained C6 activity were pooled.

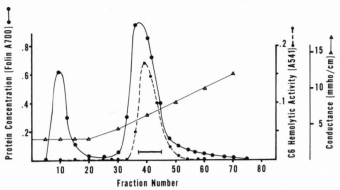

Fig. 3. Repeat of DEAE-cellulose chromatography. Column size, 2.5×50 cm. Conditions of chromatography as described in Fig. 2. Fractions 37–45 which contained C6 activity were pooled.

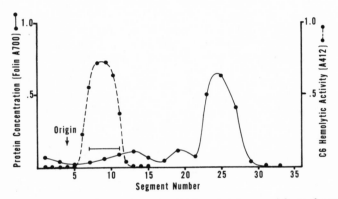

Fig. 4. Pevikon block electrophoresis of C6 containing pool from the second chromatographic step. Electrophoresis was carried out in barbital buffer, pH 8·6, $T/2 = 0.05$, for 36 hr at a potential gradient of 4 v/cm. The eluates of segments 7–11 which contained C6 activity were pooled for hydroxyapatite chromatography.

Immunochemical and gel electrophoretic examination of C6. The disc electrophoretic patterns of isolated human, rabbit and guinea pig C6 are depicted in Fig. 6.

Isolated human C6 was analyzed with various antisera to whole human serum and with monospecific antisera to γA-, γG- and γM-globulin, transferrin, albumin, C3, C4, C5, C6 and C8. Only a single line could be detected in Ouchterlony plates when either anti-whole human serum or anti-human C6 were used. The lines produced by the two antisera fused, showing that they reacted with the same antigen. None of the other antisera reacted with the isolated protein. The anti-human C6 serum gave a single line with whole human serum and this line fused without spur formation with the line of isolated human C6 (Fig. 7). An anti-rabbit C6 serum raised in a C6 deficient rabbit gave a strong precipitin

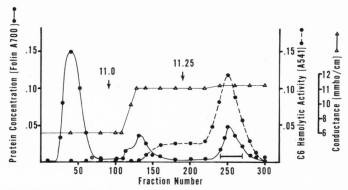

Fig. 5. Hydroxyapatite chromatography of C6 containing material from Pevikon electrophoresis. The protein was eluted in a stepwise fashion by buffers of pH 7·9 and increasing phosphate concentration, having a conductance of 8·0, 11·0 and 11·25 mmho/cm, respectively. The arrows mark the start of each successive step. Fractions 240–270 were pooled and concentrated.

reaction with isolated human C6 protein, and this antiserum produced with human and rabbit C6 a reaction of partial identity.

On immunoelectrophoresis, isolated C6 behaved like a slow β_2-globulin. The distribution of C6 hemolytic activity in the agarose gel corresponded to the location of the precipitin arc (Fig. 8). In addition to the major precipitin arc, a faint line was at times visible in the fast β-globulin region which appeared to fuse with the main arc, the latter giving rise to a spur. This related but antigenically deficient material may represent inactivated C6.

Figure 9 shows correlation of hemolytic activity and of protein on disc electrophoresis of isolated human C6. 50 μg of C6, labeled with ^{125}I, were applied to the gel, and after electrophoresis, the gel was halved and analyzed. An excellent correlation was found between the distribution of the protein, C6 hemolytic activity and radioactivity. Similar radiolabeled C6 will be used in future studies of the mechanism of action of C6.

Preparations of human C6 which on storage lost their hemolytic activity assumed a different electrophoretic behavior. On disc electrophoresis the entire protein band was shifted to a more anodal position.

Molecular weight determination. By the polyacrylamide gel electrophoresis method C6 was found to have a molecular weight of approximately 95,000 (Fig. 10), and when the molecular weight was calculated from s and D, a value of 125,000 was obtained, using a $\bar{v}$ value of 0·73. D was estimated by molecular sieve chromatography (Fig. 11) and s by sucrose density gradient ultracentrifugation (Fig. 12). Some of the molecular parameters of C6 are listed in Table 2.

Yield of C6 protein and activity. The yield of protein and hemolytic activity for preparation No. 18 is listed in Table 3. The recovery of C6 activity was approximately $\frac{1}{20}$ of the recovery of C6 protein. The reason for the apparent loss of hemolytic activity during isolation of the protein remains to be explored. In terms of C6 protein, the yield in 30 separate preparations ranged from 2–10 per cent.

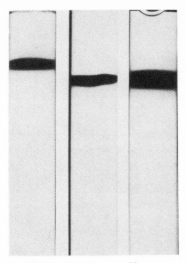

Rabbit Guinea Human
Pig

Fig. 6. Disc electrophoresis patterns of isolated C6 from human, rabbit and guinea pig serum.

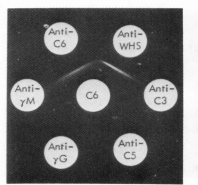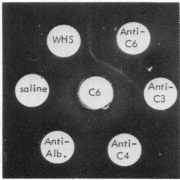

Fig. 7. Ouchterlony analysis of purified C6. 8 μg of C6 were placed into the center well. A positive reaction is seen only with anti-C6 and anti-whole human serum (Anti-WHS). As shown in the photograph at the right, the precipitin line detected by anti-C6 in human serum fused with the C6 line without spur formation. Antisera to γM, γG, C3, C4, C5 and albumin gave negative reactions.

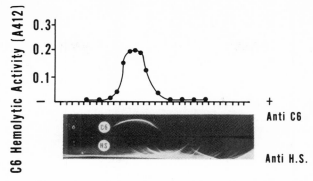

Fig. 8. Immunoelectrophoretic representation of isolated C6. For comparison, the pattern of whole human serum is shown. Electrophoresis was performed in 2 per cent agarose, veronal buffer, pH 8·6, for 2 hr at 5 v/cm. Two samples of the same C6 preparation were analyzed. One was developed with monospecific antiserum to C6, the other eluted for localization of C6 hemolytic activity. There is a good correlation between the distribution of the hemolytic activity and the localization of the precipitin arc.

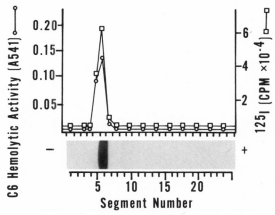

Fig. 9. Correlation between the distribution of C6 hemolytic activity, radioactivity and the protein band of purified ^{125}I-C6 after analytical polyacrylamide gel electrophoresis.

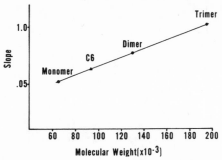

Fig. 10. Molecular weight determination by the gel electrophoresis method. The slopes were calculated from plots of the logarithm of distance of migration versus gel concentration, as outlined in the Materials and Methods section. The monomer (mol. wt. 65,000), dimer (mol. wt. 130,000) and trimer (mol. wt. 195,000) of human serum albumin were used as reference substances.

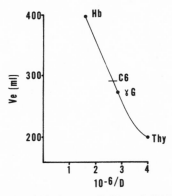

Fig. 11. Estimation of the diffusion coefficient of C6 by gel filtration on a Sephadex G-200 column. Human hemoglobin (Hb), human γG-globulin (γG) and human thyroglobulin (Thy) were used as reference substances.

Table 2. Molecular parameters of human C6

Sedimentation coefficient(s)*:	5·7S
Diffusion coefficient (D)†:	$4·0 \times 10^{-7}$ cm²/sec
Molecular weight	
s, D:	125,000
PAGE‡:	95,000
Relative electrophoretic mobility:	β_2
Serum concentration§:	60 μg/ml

*Sucrose density ultracentrifugation.
†Sephadex filtration.
‡Polyacrylamide gel electrophoresis.
§Single radial immunodiffusion.

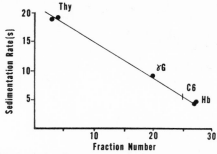

Fig. 12. Determination of sedimentation coefficient of C6 by ultracentrifugation in a linear sucrose density gradient. The data were derived from two separate experiments. The reference substances were: thyroglobulin, 19S; γG-globulin, 7S; C8, 8·5S; and hemoglobin, 4·5S.

Table 3. Recovery and yield of human C6

Preparation 18	Volume (ml)	Protein* (mg/ml)	No. of effective C6 molecules
Serum	450	60	1×10^{14}
DEAE 1	475	7	$3\cdot4 \times 10^{13}$
DEAE 2	255	5·4	$7\cdot6 \times 10^{12}$
Pevikonblock	225	0·15	$2\cdot4 \times 10^{12}$
Hydroxyapatite	5	0·16	$9\cdot6 \times 10^{10}$
Yield†		2·35%	0·1%

*Based on Folin method.

†For C6 protein based on immunochemical assay of C6 in serum (60 μg/ml).

Dose response relationship of isolated C6. Figure 13 depicts a dose response curve obtained with isolated human C6 which shows proportionality between input and number of sites formed. Using $1\cdot5 \times 10^8$ assay cells, $a - \ln (1-y)$ value of one was obtained with 300 ng of this preparation. This value varied greatly with the properties of the assay cells employed. Usually the cells contain 3000 C$\overline{4,2}$ per cell and the titrations are carried out in the presence of an excess of the remaining complement components. When the number of C$\overline{4,2}$ per cell was increased 20 times, the amount of C6 required to produce $a - \ln (1-y)$ value of unity was reduced to one-tenth. Preliminary evidence further suggests that the hemolytic efficiency of isolated C6 may be enhanced 5–6-fold either by mild treatment with reduced glutathione ($2 \times 10^{-6} M$, 2 hr, 20°) or by the presence of a small amount of highly diluted human serum (1:10,000) which *per se* produced only a negligible degree of lysis.

Quantitation of C6 in human serum. Quantitation of C6 hemolytic activity in human serum, determined under standard conditions, detected the presence of an average of $1\cdot6 \times 10^{11}$ effective molecules/ml. This amount corresponded in weight to 0·027 μg of C6/ml considering its molecular weight to be 95,000 (Table 4). By immunochemical techniques, the amount of C6 in 20 different

Table 4. Quantitation of C6 in human serum

Effective molecules per ml:	$1 \cdot 6 \times 10^{11}$
C6 protein; μg/ml	
Calculated*:	$0 \cdot 027$
Measured:	55–65
Molecules per effective	
molecule:	Approx. 3000

*Based on effective molecule titration and on a molecular weight of 95,000.

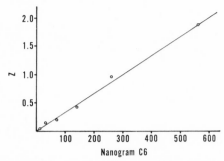

Fig. 13. Dose response for purified C6. z equals the negative natural logarithm of the proportion of unlysed cells. The number of cells was 3×10^7 per reaction mixture. A z value of unity corresponds to 63 per cent lysis.

human sera ranged between 55–65 μg/ml. The results from the two assays differ almost 3000-fold, suggesting considerable hemolytic inefficiency of C6 in serum: approximately 3000 molecules of C6 protein appear to be required for the production of one hemolytically effective molecule.

DISCUSSION

Methods for the partial purification of C6 from the serum of various species have been published previously (Nilsson and Müller-Eberhard, 1967; Rother *et al.*, 1966; Inoue and Nelson, Jr., 1965; Nilsson, 1967; Okada *et al.*, 1970; Vroon *et al.*, 1970). The present procedure is distinguished from the earlier methods in that it allows the preparation of C6 as a highly homogeneous protein. As such, it could be demonstrated by disc electrophoresis and immunoelectrophoresis. It was characterized as a β-globulin with a molecular weight of 95,000 or 125,000 depending on the method used. Its concentration in normal human serum is 55–65 μg/ml. Monospecific antisera were produced in normal and genetically C6 deficient rabbits, and using an anti-rabbit C6 made in a C6 deficient animal, a close immunochemical relationship could be demonstrated between human C6 and the rabbit analogue.

Largely unexplained at present remains the loss of hemolytic activity which almost all preparations sustained during the hydroxyapatite step, by which final purification of the protein is achieved. The possibility was raised, therefore, that a heretofore unrecognized complement factor or cofactor of C6 is removed during this step. In fact, less highly purified preparations were found to be more active than the purest preparations. The enhancement of isolated C6 by a very small amount of human serum, which *per se* was virtually inactive in the C6 assay, would tend to favor the missing-factor hypothesis. On the other hand, the observed enhancing effect of mild treatment of isolated C6 with reduced glutathione suggests an alternative explanation. It is conceivable that glutathione removed metal ions from free sulfhydryl groups which might be essential for the expression of full hemolytic activity. That sulfhydryl groups may have relevant functions in the complement reaction has been demonstrated previously for C2 and C3 (Polley and Müller-Eberhard, 1969). More work is needed to distinguish between these possibilities.

Isolated C6 with reduced hemolytic activity as compared to C6 in serum closely resembles the latter in electrophoretic mobility, *s*-rate and immunochemical properties. In contrast, hemolytically inactive C6 exhibits a distinctly faster mobility on polyacrylamide gel electrophoresis.

C6 assumed particular significance when it was shown that biological activity other than cytolytic and bactericidal activity is generated by the complement system (Ward *et al.*, 1966). A high molecular weight product of C5, C6 and C7 was identified as a chemotactic factor for polymorphonuclear leukocytes. Although the precise nature of the active product remains to be defined, the observation was confirmed by Lachmann *et al.* (1970) who utilized the reactive hemolysis system in their work.

An inherited complement defect in rabbits, first observed by Rother and Rother (1961), could be delineated as an isolated C6 deficiency (Rother *et al.*, 1966). The animals are unable to synthesize C6 protein and can therefore produce antibody to rabbit C6 when injected with rabbit serum or isolated rabbit C6. The deficient animals are difficult to breed and the impression prevails that their survival chances are diminished (Rother and Rother, 1961). Their serum does sustain phagocytosis *in vitro*, but it lacks bactericidal and cytolytic activity. Recently, Johnson and Ward (1971) found a requirement of C6 for the detoxification of bacterial endotoxins by serum. A marked impairment in the detoxifying capacity was found in C6 deficient rabbit serum, which could be completely corrected by addition of isolated human C6 prepared in our laboratory.

The present work on C6 led to the initial recognition of a previously unknown physiological function of this protein. Blood obtained from C6 deficient rabbits was found to have a coagulation defect without lacking any of the classical clotting factors (Zimmerman *et al.*, 1971). Addition of physiological amounts of human or rabbit C6 isolated according to the above described procedure fully normalized coagulation of the deficient blood. None of the classical clotting factors were found in preparations of isolated human C6. Participation of C6 in the normal coagulation mechanism of human blood was revealed by the demonstration of the consumption of 10–15 per cent of C6 during coagulation.

The availability of highly purified C6 and of monospecific antiserum will aid the delineation of the molecular events underlying the various biological manifestations of C6.

REFERENCES

Andrews P. (1965) *Biochem. J.* **96**, 595.
Arroyave C. M. and Müller-Eberhard H. J. (1970) *Fedn. Proc.* **29**, 434.
Davis B. J. (1964) *Ann. N.Y. Acad. Sci.* **121**, 404.
Folin O. and Ciocalteu U. (1927) *J. biol. Chem.* **73**, 627.
Götze O. and Müller-Eberhard H. J. (1970) *J. exp. Med.* **132**, 898.
Goudie R. B., Horne C. H. and Wilkinson P. C. (1966) *Lancet* **ii**, 1124.
Hadding U. and Müller-Eberhard H. J. (1969) *Immunology* **16**, 719.
Hedrick J. L. and Smith A. J. (1968) *Arch. Biochem. Biophys.* **126**, 155.
Inoue K. and Nelson R. A., Jr. (1965) *J. Immun.* **95**, 355.
Johnson K. J. and Ward P. A. (1971) *Fedn. Proc.* **30**, 356.
Kabat E. A. and Mayer M. M. (1961) *Experimental Immunochemistry*, p. 133. Thomas, Springfield, Ill.
Kunkel H. G. (1960) *The Plasma Proteins* (Edited by Putnam F. W.), p. 279. Academic Press, New York.
Lachmann P. J. (1970) *Protides of the Biological Fluids* (Edited by Peeters H.), p. 301. Pergamon Press, Oxford and New York.
Lachmann P. J., Kay A. B. and Thompson R. A. (1970) *Immunology* **19**, 895.
Mancini G., Carbonara A. O. and Heremans J. F. (1965) *Immunochemistry* **2**, 325.
Manni J. A. and Müller-Eberhard H. J. (1969) *J. exp. Med.* **130**, 1145.
McConahey P. J. and Dixon F. J. (1966) *Int. Arch. Allergy Appl. Immunol.* **29**, 185.
Müller-Eberhard H. J. (1960) *Scand. J. Clin. Lab. Invest.* **12**, 33.
Müller-Eberhard H. J. and Biro C. E. (1963) *J. exp. Med.* **118**, 447.
Nelson R. A., Jr. and Biro C. E. (1968) *Immunology* **14**, 527.
Nelson R. A., Jr., Jensen J., Gigli I. and Tamura N. (1966) *Immunochemistry* **3**, 111.
Nilsson U. R. (1967) *Acta Path. Microbiol. Scand.* **70**, 469.
Nilsson U. R. and Müller-Eberhard H. J. (1965) *J. exp. Med.* **122**, 277.
Nilsson U. R. and Müller-Eberhard H. J. (1967) *Immunology* **13**, 101.
Okada H., Mayumi M., Mukojima T., Sekine T. and Torisu M. (1970) *Immunology* **18**, 493.
Ouchterlony Ö. (1967) *Handbook of Experimental Immunology* (Edited by Weir D. M.), p. 655. Blackwell Scientific Publications, Oxford and Edinburgh.
Polley M. J. and Müller-Eberhard H. J. (1968) *J. exp. Med.* **128**, 533.
Polley M. J. and Müller-Eberhard H. J. (1969) *J. Immun.* **102**, 1339.
Rother U. and Rother K. (1961) *Z. Immunitatsforsch.* **121**, 224.
Rother K., Rother U., Müller-Eberhard H. J. and Nilsson U. R. (1966) *J. exp. Med.* **124**, 773.
Scheidegger J. J. (1955) *Int. Arch. Allergy Appl. Immunol.* **33**, 11.
Tiselius A., Hjerten S. and Levin Ö. (1956) *Arch. Biochem. Biophys.* **65**, 132.
Vroon D. H., Schultz D. R. and Zarco R. M. (1970) *Immunochemistry* **7**, 43.
Ward P. A., Cochrane C. G. and Müller-Eberhard H. J. (1966) *Immunology* **11**, 141.
Zimmerman T. S. and Müller-Eberhard H. J. (1971) *J. exp. Med.* (Submitted).
Zimmerman T. S., Arroyave C. M. and Müller-Eberhard H. J. (1971) *J. exp. Med.* (Submitted).

Properties

FUNCTION AND PHYSICAL PROPERTIES OF TWO DISTINCT FORMS OF THE FIRST COMPONENT OF GUINEA PIG COMPLEMENT*

JAMES J. THOMPSON† and LOUIS G. HOFFMANN

Abstract—Both types of partially purified guinea pig Cl (first component of complement), prepared by solubility chromatography at low ionic strength and pH 7·5, are obtained in activated form. In contrast to Cl in whole serum, both produce linear dose response curves. The more soluble of the two, Type A, fails to bind to antigen–antibody complexes, is physically heterogeneous, and is smaller in size than the other, Type B. The evidence suggests that Type A, which cannot be detected in whole serum, arises by degradation during purification.

INTRODUCTION

A recent report from this laboratory[2] described the isolation of two types of Cl‡ from guinea pig serum; one of these (Type A) is soluble at pH 7·5, ionic strength $\mu = 0.0105$, the other (Type B) is not. The study whose results are described in the present report was undertaken to characterize these two forms of Cl both functionally and physically. We wished to ascertain whether one or both Types of Cl are enzymatically active or in the proenzyme state found in serum[15]; what the dose response of each type is, and whether they act independently of each other when added together in an assay system containing EAC4 and C2; whether one or both forms can bind to sensitized sheep erythrocytes (EA); whether one or both originate as artefacts during isolation; and what, if any, relationship exists between these two forms of guinea pig Cl and the subcomponents, Clq, Clr, and Cls, recognized in the human C system.

MATERIALS AND METHODS

Preparation of diluents, complement, EA and EAC4 (high multiplicity) followed the procedures of Hoffmann, McKenzie, and Mayer[3]. Cell blanks in Cl assays were treated by the revised method of Hoffmann[4]. Veronal buffers of varying ionic strength were prepared by the method of Rapp and Borsos[5].

p-Nitrophenylethyl benzyl phosphonate (PNPEBP)[9] was the generous gift of Dr. E. L. Becker. A 5 mM stock solution was prepared in dry acetone and diluted as needed.

*Supported by NIH Research Grant No. AI-06436, NSF Research Grant No. GB-7881, and a General Research Support Grant to the University of Iowa, College of Medicine. A preliminary report has been given to the American Association of Immunologists, April 1968, Atlantic City, New Jersey.

†Pre-Doctoral Fellow of the NIH. Part of this work was presented by J. J. T. to the Graduate College, University of Iowa, in partial fulfillment of the requirements for the M.S.

‡The nomenclature in this report follows that set forth in *W.H.O. Bull.* **39**, 935 (1968).

Partially purified C1 was prepared by solubility chromatography at pH 5·6, and Type A and Type B C1 were resolved by solubility chromatography at pH 7·5 as described by Hoffmann[10].

C2 used to study fluid phase destruction by C1 was prepared by ion exchange column chromatography according to Borsos, *et al.*[11]. All other C2 was prepared by solubility chromatography in concentrated $(NH_4)_2SO_4$ as described by Hoffmann and McGivern[12], followed by 3 cycles of gel filtration on Sephadex G-200.

Routine C1 assays were performed according to the method given by Hoffmann *et al.*[3], except for C1 in serum, which requires activation[15]. For this purpose, 1·0 ml of EAC4 ($2·5 \times 10^8$/ml) was incubated with 1·0 ml of a serum dilut on for 3 hr at 37°C. We then added 1·0 ml of an appropriate C2 dilution (the same amount as used in other assays), and proceeded as described earlier[3]. In a few of the experiments, these procedures were altered for reasons and in ways to be indicated in each particular case.

C2 was assayed by the method of Mayer and Miller[7] except that the reaction was carried out at $\mu = 0·065$ and $EAC\overline{1}, 4$ was prepared by adding sufficient Type B C1 to EAC4 (10^9/ml) to give 150 SFU of C1 per EAC4. C2 results were analyzed by the dose response model of Hoffmann and Meier[8].

We employed centrifugation in sucrose density gradients to compare the molecular sizes of C1 in whole serum and of Types A and B. The sucrose solutions and the samples contained 10 mM TRIS-HCl, 70 mM NaCl, and 0·5 mM $CaCl_2$, and were adjusted to pH 7·0 at room temperature. Linear 10–30% (w/v) sucrose (Density Gradient Grade, Mann Research Labs., New York, N. Y.) concentration gradients were formed with a Spinco gradient pump; 200 μl samples containing no sucrose were layered on top of the gradients. Centrifugation took place for 8·5 hr in a Spinco SW-56 rotor at 408,000 **g** (at r_{max}) at a rotor temperature setting of 0°C; a Spinco Model L4 centrifuge was used. Hog thyroglobulin (Mann Research Labs., New York, N.Y.), rabbit γG immunoglobulin (Immunology, Inc., Glen Ellyn, Illinois), and crystalline bovine serum albumin (Pentex Inc., Kankakee, Illinois) were employed as markers.

After centrifugation was complete, we removed the tubes to an ice bath and fractionated them in a cold room at 2–5°C. A 46 per cent sucrose solution, containing the same salt concentrations as the gradient and 0·01 per cent Bromophenol Blue as an optical marker, was pumped into the bottom of the tube through a needle. The gradient solution emerging from the top of the tube was passed through a conductivity cell and through a flow-through spectrophotometer cuvette with a 10 mm light path, which are part of the system for fractionating chromatographic effluents described earlier[10]; 3 drop fractions were collected into tubes containing $2·5 \times 10^8$ EA in 0·5 ml of mannitol-buffer. The flow rate for this operation was adjusted to about 5 drops /min.

The conductivity cell, which had a cell constant of 0·704 cm^{-1}, was connected to a conductivity bridge (LKB Conductolyzer) capable of producing a recorder output proportional to the impedance across the conductivity cell. Since sucrose affects the dielectric constant of its solutions and since the salt concentrations are uniform, recording impedence changes is tantamount to recording capacitance changes across the conductivity cell; these changes reflect changes in sucrose concentration. The recorder traces were converted to sucrose concentration curves on the basis of a calibration plot.

The sucrose solution with its dye marker, which was used to displace the gradients from the centrifuge tubes, also provided a convenient way to measure dead volume between conductivity cell, spectrophotometer cuvette, and fraction collector. The recorder traces were shifted appropriately to coincide with the activity curves on the basis of these measurements.

C1 activity in samples derived from whole serum or Type B C1 was assayed after transferring the C1 from the EA to 2.5×10^8 EAC4 according to the method of Borsos and Rapp[13]. C1 in samples from Type A C1 was assayed by the method referred to above[3]; as will be shown below, Type A C1 does not bind to cells, and therefore transfer assays were unnecessary in this case.

RESULTS

Origin of type A and type B C1

Since Hoffmann isolated Type A and Type B C1 from a partially purified preparation of C1 as the starting material, the question of pre-existing multiple forms of C1 in whole serum remained open. Figure 1 depicts results obtained by solubility chromatography at pH 7·5 and low ionic strength of 10·0 ml of pooled guinea pig serum. Recovery is 5–10 per cent of the activity originally present. Virtually all of the C1 activity that is recovered is in the Type B peak with traces of Type A present. However, the serum C1 inhibitor should migrate with the

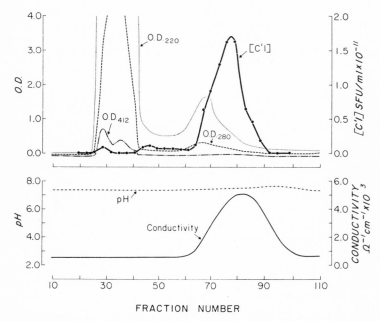

Fig. 1. Solubility chromatography of guinea pig serum at pH 7·5 and low ionic strength.

102

'soluble' protein peak containing Type A Cl[14]; therefore, the presence of Type A Cl is not rigorously excluded.

Another possibility raised by the existence of multiple forms of Cl concerns interconversion between these types: Does one form represent a functionally active degradation product of the other? Figure 2 shows experiments designed to answer this question. The Cl prepared by solubility chromatography of 200 ml of serum at pH 5·6 and low ionic strength was concentrated to 15 ml and divided into two equal portions. The first portion was kept strictly at 0°C and analyzed by solubility chromatography at pH 7·5. The Type B Cl peak contained most of the Cl activity although Type A Cl was present. The second portion of partially purified Cl was heated at 37°C for 15 min, cooled, and then chromato-

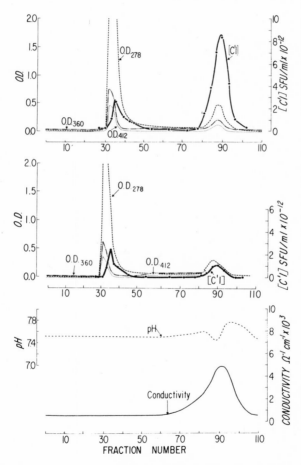

Fig. 2. Solubility chromatography of partially purified Cl. Top panel: Cl sample kept at 0°C. Middle panel: Cl sample heated for 15 min at 37°C. Lower panel: pH and conductivity for above runs.

graphed under the same conditions as the first portion. Type B activity declines significantly, but Type A activity remains virtually intact.

This activity loss could be due either to direct inactivation of Type B C1, or to its conversion to Type A, which might then lose activity in turn, resulting in a steady state with respect to Type A activity. Two experiments were designed to discriminate between these alternatives. Table 1 shows that after heating each C1 preparation separately for 15 min at 37°C, Type B C1 retains activity only if it is heated in diluted form; Type A maintains full activity in either case. This result suggests that Type B C1 loses activity directly.

Table 1. The effect of heating on C1 hemolytic activity

Treatment	Percent C1 remaining Type A	Type B
15 min, 0°C undiluted	(100)	(100)
15 min, 37°C undiluted	93·5	55·4
15 min, 37°C diluted 1 : 26	105	95·0

To determine whether the C1 activity which remains in a Type B preparation after heating is still Type B, a heated sample of Type B C1 was analyzed by solubility chromatography at pH 7·5. All the residual activity emerged in the position corresponding to Type B.

Reaction of Type A and Type B C1 in the complement system

Dose response and conditions for assay. Figure 3 depicts the dose response of C1 in whole guinea pig serum, obtained with activation of C1 to $\overline{\text{C1}}$ by incubation of whole serum dilutions with EAC4 at 37°C for 3 hr. Although the dose response is linear through most of its range, it is convex to the abscissa near the origin.

To study the dose response of Type A and Type B C1, we changed the reaction volume in the initial steady state mixture. Each tube received 1·0 ml EAC4, $2·5 \times 10^8$/ml, 1·0 ml C2, 1·0 ml of a given dilution of Type A C1 or buffer, and 1·0 ml of a given dilution of Type B C1 or buffer. The remainder of the assay was carried out as usual[3].

The results, shown in Fig. 4, demonstrate that the dose response data of isolated Type A and Type B C1 are linear and extrapolate to the origin. The figure also shows that the dose response of a mixture of Type A and Type B C1 is additive: The sum of the slopes of the individual dose response lines equals the slope of the combined dose response.

To study the effect of ionic strength on the activities of both types of C1, we found it necessary to change the assay system because centrifugation of $\text{EAC}\overline{1}$, 4, $\overline{2}$ at very low ionic strength gave hyperagglutinated cells which could not be resuspended in C'EDTA until incubation for about 5 min at 37°C. Erratic results occurred, presumably due to variable decay of $\text{SAC}\overline{1}$, 4, $\overline{2}$ during this

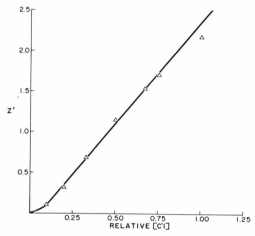

Fig. 3. Dose response of Cl in guinea pig serum; z' = corrected average number of $SAC\overline{1,4,2}$ per cell.

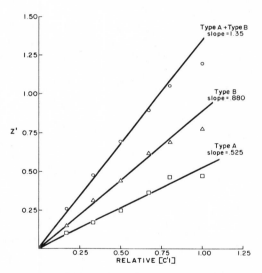

Fig. 4. Dose response of Type A and Type B Cl; z' = corrected average number of $SAC\overline{1,4,2}$ per cell.

period. Therefore, we used a Cl assay similar to that of Borsos and Rapp[6] for experiments on the effect of ionic strength. In this assay system, $8\cdot33 \times 10^7$ EAC4 were suspended in $0\cdot5$ ml of an appropriate dilution of C2 and $0\cdot5$ ml of a Cl dilution. The C2 and Cl dilutions were made in buffer of the ionic strength to be examined. After incubation at 30°C for 30 min, the tubes were transferred to 0°C, and 9 ml of cold C diluted 1/62·5 in EDTA-buffer (C'EDTA) were added.

After incubation at 37°C for 90 min, the tubes were centrifuged and the optical densities of the supernatant fluids measured at 412 nm.

Ionic strength profoundly affects the level of the steady state as demonstrated in Fig. 5. Constant amounts of C1 were added to each of the tubes, but the ionic strength of the mixtures was varied. Both C1 types show a skewed, bell-shaped response, but the Type A activity curve is displaced slightly toward lower ionic strengths when compared to the Type B curve.

Binding to antigen–antibody complexes. One ml of EA at two times the desired final cell concentration was mixed with $1·0$ ml of a C1 dilution containing $1·17 \times 10^9$ SFU of Type A or $1·78 \times 10^9$ SFU of Type B. After reaction for 15 min at 30°C, the tubes were centrifuged at room temperature, and the supernatant fluids analyzed for free C1. The difference between this value and the total C1, as assayed in control tubes receiving no cells, was assumed to represent bound C1. The binding reaction was done at $\mu = 0·065$ for Type B C1 and at $\mu = 0·037$ for Type A on the basis of the finding that these ionic strengths are optimal for the activity of the respective C1 species (see Fig. 5). Free C1 was assayed in both cases, however, at $\mu = 0·065$.

The results are shown in Fig. 6 for both types of C1. Most Type B C1 can be bound to EA if the cell concentration is high enough. Type A shows no significant binding at any cell concentration up to 10^9/ml. Similar results were obtained with EAC4 by examining both the cells and the supernatant fluids. C1 binding to EAC4 was also studied in the presence of C2, with the same outcome.

Activation state. Guinea pig C1 may exist as the hemolytically inactive precursor form C1 in serum but is hemolytically active $\overline{C1}$ upon isolation[15]. $\overline{C1}$ can be distinguished from C1 by three criteria: kinetics of $SA\overline{C1},4$ formation, fluid

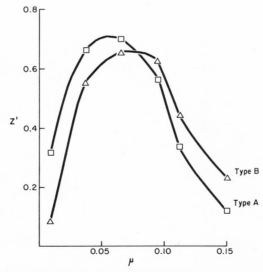

Fig. 5. Ionic strength dependence of the steady state reaction system in the presence of limited C1; z' = corrected average number of $SA\overline{C1},4,\overline{2}$ per cell.

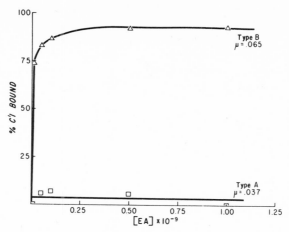

Fig. 6. Binding of C1 to EA. Cell concentration is in cells/ml.

phase destruction of C2, and inhibition by PNPEBP, which acts in a manner analogous to diisopropyl fluorophosphate[9]. We examined both types of C1 by all three criteria; the results show that both types are in the activated form.

Since Type A C1 does not bind to EAC4, $SAC\overline{1}$, 4 formation cannot be studied with this form of C1. Instead, we followed the formation of $SAC\overline{1}$, 4, $\overline{2}$ kinetically after addition of each type of C1 to a mixture of EAC4 and C2 at $\mu = 0.065$. The kinetics of $SAC\overline{1}$, 4, $\overline{2}$ formation were probably paced by the reaction of EAC4 with C1 since in our experiment a large amount of C2 was present.

One ml of an appropriate C1 dilution was added to a flask containing 2.5×10^9 EAC4 and 600 units[8] of C2 in a final volume of 30.0 ml, which had been warmed to 30°C. Samples of 1.0 ml of the reaction mixture were removed during incubation at the same temperature and added to 4.0 ml of ice-cold veronal buffer containing 10 mM EDTA. The sample tubes were centrifuged at 0°C within 10 min of the time of withdrawal, and the cells were resuspended in 2.0 ml of C'EDTA diluted 1/62.5, and incubated 90 min at 37°C. At the end of this period, 6.5 ml of 0.15 M NaCl were added to each tube, the tubes were centrifuged, and the O. D. of the supernatant fluids was measured at 412 nm. The usual calculations were performed, and the results were corrected for lysis ('CBC') in a control flask which had received no C1 [4].

Figure 7 shows the results of this experiment. With Type B C1, a steady state with respect to $SAC\overline{1},4,\overline{2}$ concentration is achieved in less than 30 min, in close agreement with the observation of Borsos et al.[15] for purified $C\overline{1}$. The reaction with Type A C1 is decidedly slower, but still considerably faster than the formation of $SAC\overline{1},4$ by EAC4 and C1 supplied by unfractionated serum[15]. A steady state is maintained for a shorter period than with Type B C1; this probably reflects faster depletion of C2 from the fluid phase, which is to be expected when most of the C1 is not cell-bound.

Fluid phase destruction of C2 by C1 was measured as follows: To 6.5 ml of

107

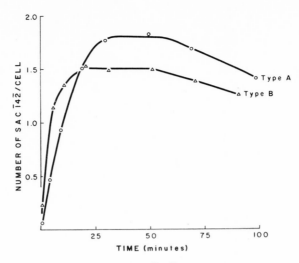

Fig. 7. Kinetics of SAC$\overline{1}$,4,$\overline{2}$ formation at 30°C.

mannitol buffer ($\mu = 0.065$) were added 2·5 ml of a C2 dilution containing about 3.6×10^8 SFU/ml. After incubation for 10 min at 30°C, 1·0 ml of a C1 dilution was added. One-milliliter samples of this mixture were taken at various times, diluted into 4·0 ml of ice-cold mannitol buffer ($\mu = 0.065$) and assayed for residual C2. We determined the initial reaction rates by inspection of the plots of C2 remaining in the reaction mixture against time.

The destruction of C2 by both C1 types occurs with no detectable lag. The initial rates of destruction are directly proportional to C1 concentration as shown in Fig. 8. Thus, C1 of both types is enzymatically active and conforms to one of the Michaelis–Menten assumptions; no deviations associated with

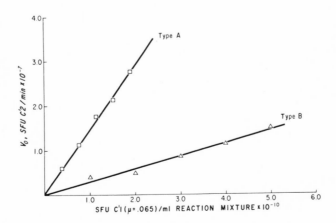

Fig. 8. Fluid phase inactivation of C2 by C1.

108

conversion C1 to C$\overline{1}$ occur. When the SFU input of C1 for both types is computed from C1 assays made at $\mu = 0.065$, Type A C1 appears five times more efficient in C2 destruction than Type B.

We studied the kinetics of C1 inactivation by PNPEBP by adding 0.20 ml of a 5 mM solution of PNPEBP in acetone to 2.5 ml of mannitol buffer at 30°C, followed by 2.5 ml of a C1 dilution containing 1.47×10^{10} SFU/ml for Type A, 1.07×10^{10} SFU/ml for Type B, and 5.65×10^{9} SFU/ml for serum. At various times, samples of 1.0 ml were diluted 50-fold in ice-cold mannitol buffer, and assayed for residual C1. Whole serum samples were assayed with activation for 3.0 hr at 37°C by incubation with EAC4. Control tubes were treated as described above, except that each tube received 0.20 ml of acetone containing no PNPEBP.

Figure 9 shows the sensitivity of C1 to inhibition by $2 \times 10^{-4}\,M$ PNPEBP. C1 present in whole guinea pig serum resists such treatment; both Type A and Type B C1 are readily inactivated under the same conditions. Type A appears 1.3 times more sensitive to PNPEBP inhibition than Type B. Deviations from first order kinetics become significant after 15 min, probably because the inhibitor hydrolyzes spontaneously.

Physical studies

Attempts to characterize and purify both types of C1 by gel filtration on Sephadex G-200 or on agarose (Sepharose 4B) columns in a variety of solvents were uniformly unsuccessful because of low or nonexistent recoveries. With regard to Sephadex, our experience coincides with that of Linscott[16]. Ultracentrifigation on sucrose density gradients was therefore chosen to define the relative molecular sizes of the two forms of C1.

We examined six lots of Type B C1 and five of Type A. Control samples of Type B C1, which were not centrifuged but maintained at 0°C for the duration

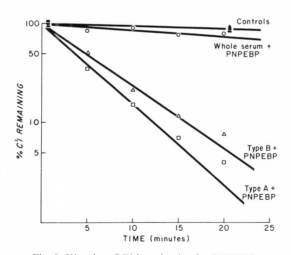

Fig. 9. Kinetics of C1 inactivation by PNPEBP.

of the experiment (*ca.* 36 hr), showed more than 90 per cent inactivation; additional activity was lost in the centrifuged samples. No major loss of activity occurred in Type A C1. The interpretations of the results of the centrifuge experiments rests on the assumption that the Type B C1 activity surviving this extensive inactivation is a representative sample of the activity present originally. Since this assumption is untestable, our conclusions based on these experiments must remain tentative. The results obtained for Type B C1 were consistent, and typical data are shown in Fig. 10, panel A. The results for Type A C1 varied considerably between the different lots examined; the data obtained for two of them are shown in Fig. 10, panels B and C. The sucrose concentration corresponding to the position of the peak of each marker protein is indicated by the appropriately labeled arrow in Fig. 10. Under the conditions of centrifugation employed here, bovine serum albumin and rabbit γG immunoglobulin are not resolved; therefore, the position of the former is not indicated.

The active material in Type B C1 sedimented as a single zone with a suggestion of heterogeneity at its leading edge. Its position was slightly ahead of that of thyroglobulin, suggesting a sedimentation coefficient of about 20 S. Each of the six different preparations of Type B C1 that were examined gave the same result.

The sedimentation patterns for Type A C1 provide conclusive evidence for the heterogeneity of these preparations. In Fig. 10, panel B, which represents results obtained in the same centrifuge run as those shown in panel A, most of the activity sediments with approximately 19 S, with a less prominent peak at 7 S. Although the major C1 fraction in this preparation has the same size as Type B C1, it is functionally different from Type B: The C1 assays on fractions from this tube were performed without transfer and thus represent C1 activity which is not bound to EA at $\mu = 0.065$.

Data for another preparation of Type A C1, obtained in a separate centrifuge run, are shown in Fig. 10, panel C, to illustrate the differences in size distribution that occur between preparations of Type A C1. A different size distribution was obtained for each of the five Type A C1 preparations examined; repeated centrifuge runs on some of the preparations produced consistent results. Most of the material absorbing or scattering light is confined to the very top of the gradient, indicating that the turbidity observed in these preparations is mostly due to lipid.

DISCUSSION

Each of the two C1 types has a linear dose response relation extrapolating to the origin, and behaves independently of the other in the assay system.

The lack of cooperative or inhibitory interactions between the two species, as indicated by the additivity of the dose responses, suggests that each C1 type is functionally independent of the other. In contrast, cooperative effects have been demonstrated among the subunits of human C1. C1q, C1r, or C1s alone gave no hemolytic activity; C1r + C1s gave some activity when assayed with EAC4, but full activity required the simultaneous presence of all three factors [18]. More recent work suggests that C1s is hemolytically active without C1r or C1q[19]. With respect to its activity in the hemolytic system, human C1s corresponds closely to our Type A C1.

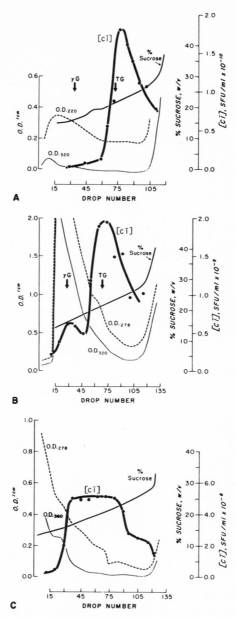

Fig. 10. Sucrose density gradient centrifugation of C1. Panel A: Type B C1. Panels B and C: Type A C1. Panels A and B represent data obtained in a single run; panel C is taken from a different run. The positions in the gradient of rabbit γG immunoglobulin (γG) and of hog thyroglobulin (TG) are indicated by appropriately labeled vertical arrows.

The reactivity of both Type A and Type B C1 without activation in the conventional C1 assay system suggests that they are functionally $\overline{\text{C1}}$. Three different lines of evidence prove that this is indeed the case. (i) The kinetics of $\text{SAC}\overline{1},4,\overline{2}$ formation show that maximal activity results soon after mixing of C1 with EAC4; the gradual appearance of $\text{SAC}\overline{1},4,\overline{2}$ associated with activation of bound C1 to $\overline{\text{C1}}$ does not occur. (ii) PNPEBP inactivates both C1 types readily but whole serum C1 resists such treatment. It might be argued that the apparent inability of PNPEBP to inactivate C1 in serum could be due to hydrolysis of the reagent by a hypothetical serum esterase; this is unlikely in view of the earlier studies of Levine[27] and Becker[28] on the effect of diisopropyl fluorophosphate (DFP) on C1 in serum. These studies showed that C1 in serum is inactivated by DFP only in the presence of EA, which causes conversion of C1 to $\overline{\text{C1}}$; an esterase capable of hydrolysing phosphonates would have had the same effect in either case. (iii) Both C1 types behave as enzymes by catalyzing the fluid phase destruction of substrate (C2) and obey the classical laws of enzyme kinetics with respect to the effect of enzyme concentration on initial rate.

Our ionic strength studies show that increasing the ionic strength decreases the apparent titer of both Type A and Type B C1. At least three effects may contribute to the decrease: (i) Dissociating C1 from the cell[13] may decrease the number of sites yielding $\text{SAC}4,\overline{2}$ even though the C1 may be cycling among more sites. (ii) The K_m of the C2 fixation reaction increases with increasing ionic strength[3]. (iii) Substrate (SAC4,2) concentration decreases with increasing ionic strength. Sitomer et al.[20] found reversible binding of C2 to EAC4 to reach a maximum at about $\mu = 0.04$ and to decrease with increasing ionic strength.

The Type A ionic strength-activity curve is similar in shape to that of the Type B curve but is displaced slightly toward lower ionic strength. This displacement of the Type A curve with respect to the Type B curve may reflect solubility differences of the two C1 types. Type A remains active at ionic strengths where Type B loses activity; this result is consistent with the results obtained by solubility chromatography at pH 7·5. At very low ionic strength both species probably precipitate; this behavior manifests itself in the curves for both C1 types at very low ionic strength where steady state activity falls off markedly.

We have obtained three distinct measures of the biological activity of each type of C1: (i) hemolytic activity in the catalysis of $\text{SAC}4,\overline{2}$ formation from the reversible complex[20] SAC4,2; (ii) enzymatic activity in the fluid phase inactivation of C2; and (iii) irreversible inhibition by the phosphonate ester PNPEBP. Because we were unable to demonstrate binding of Type A C1 to EA or EAC4, we attribute its hemolytic effectiveness to transitory interaction with the substrate complex SAC4,2. This can have two opposite effects on the hemolytic efficiency, i.e., the ratio of SFU to molecules, of Type A C1: (i) Because the interaction is transitory, the turnover rate at which the enzyme cycles from one molecular SAC4,2 complex to the next, and thus the hemolytic efficiency, may be increased; and (ii) the number of effective collisions of enzyme which substrate may be reduced. The results of the ionic strength experiments with Type B C1, whose binding is reduced at $\mu > 0.065$, indicate that the depressing effect predominates. We would therefore expect the hemolytic efficiency of Type A C1 to be less than that of Type B and certainly less than 1·0. In the absence of purified preparations of both types of C1, an absolute measure of their hemolytic efficiencies is impossible.

The results of our PNPEBP inactivation studies, which are independent of the hemolytic efficiency because pseudo-first order conditions prevailed with respect to C1 concentration, indicate that the catalytic site in Type A C1 is more accessible, at least to small molecules, than in Type B. Another possibility, viz., a change in the conformation of the catalytic site itself, seems less likely to us, although it cannot be excluded on the basis of present data.

The initial rate of C2 inactivation by Type A C1 is 5 times greater than that of Type B on the basis of hemolytic activity measurements. Three possible explanations, which are not mutually exclusive, may be advanced for this difference: (i) It could be due to greater accessibility of the catalytic site of Type A C1 to C2, as compared to that of Type B; the results of the PNPEBP experiment suggest that this is the case, but cannot be applied quantitatively in view of the enormous difference in molecular size between the two reagents. (ii) The difference in C2 inactivation rates could also be due to a difference in size between the two types of C1 if the inactivation were diffusion controlled; but this seems unlikely. (iii) It is more reasonable to ascribe at least part of the difference in apparent C2 inactivation rates to a difference in hemolytic efficiency, since hemolytic activity is the basis of comparison. By attributing the entire difference to this cause alone, we can place an upper limit of 5 on the ratio of hemolytic efficiencies of Type B to Type A C1. This estimate rests on the assumption that the enzymatically active sites of Types A and B C1 react with C2 in identical fashion; although this assumption appears reasonable to us, we do not have experimental support for it.

Nagaki and Stroud[19] have reported functional studies on purified preparations of the human sub-component, C1s, which indicated a remarkable similarity in biological properties between human C1s and our Type A C1. However, the implicit suggestion that Type A C1 represents a guinea pig analog of human C1s must be discarded in the light of our ultracentrifugal studies on the size of Type A C1, which clearly indicate heterogeneity.

This heterogeneity strongly favors the concept that Type A C1 is the product of degradation which occurred in the process of purification. The apparent absence of Type A C1 from whole guinea pig serum is consistent with this interprepation. However, this conclusion must remain tentative in view of our failure to reproduce Type A C1 formation by incubating a partially purified C1 preparation at 37°C; it is possible that the conditions chosen for this experiment were not appropriate, but we have not investigated this further. That Type A C1 production might occur under different conditions is suggested by our observation that on prolonged storage at −65°C, a Type B C1 preparation lost part of its activity and part of its ability to bind to EA; solubility chromatography at low ionic strength and pH 7·5 demonstrated the presence of a significant amount of Type A C1 in this preparation. The failure of Type A C1 to bind to EA suggests that it is a fragment of C1 lacking the analog of the human subunit C1q.

The observed heterogeneity of Type A, but not of Type B, C1 cannot be due to ionic strength dependent dissociation into subunits of the type described by

Colten *et al.*[22], for several reasons. First, the ionic strength at which all samples were examined was 0·08. The data of Colten *et al.*[22] indicate that their partially purified guinea pig $C\overline{1}$ preparation sediments at 19 S at $\mu = 0·065$, and at 17 S at $\mu = 0·15$; at $\mu = 0·08$, dissociation should therefore be minimal, and certainly not sufficient to account for material sedimenting at about 7 S. We chose $\mu = 0·08$, rather than $\mu = 0·065$, to avoid aggregation which might occur under conditions where Type B C1 approaches its solubility limit. Second, since both Type A and Type B C1 were centrifuged under the same conditions, any dissociation should have affected both preparations to the same extent; hence, dissociation cannot be advanced as an explanation for the difference between the two types of preparation.

It might be argued that Type A C1 arose by dissociation into subunits during preparation. This argument is incompatible with the observed physical heterogeneity of Type A C1; if it were a subunit it should have a defined molecular size. Furthermore, the conditions of solubility chromatography at low ionic strength and pH 7·5 favor association rather than dissociation of subunits: Conductivity measurements indicate that the C1 fraction is applied to the column at $\mu \approx 0·22$; but as it migrates into the gradient, its ionic strength decreases at the rate of 0·012/hr. Since this change is being imposed on a highly concentrated C1 solution, it seems likely that association of subunits, if any, would occur fast enough to keep up with the change in equilibrium resulting from the reduction in ionic strength.

Our estimate of the sedimentation coefficient of purified Type B C1 at $\mu = 0·08$ agrees with that obtained by Colten *et al.*[22] for guinea pig $C\overline{1}$, purified by a different procedure and examined at $\mu = 0·065$. In most respects, therefore, our Type B $C\overline{1}$ preparations resemble partially purified guinea pig $C\overline{1}$ obtained by other precipitation methods. These preparations differ in two ways from native C1 as it occurs in serum, viz., in dose response and in activation state. Since our studies indicate that fragmentation of C1 occurs during purification even under conditions of minimal contact between the precipitated C1 and the supernatnat fluid[10], it seems relevant to raise the question whether the observed differences between Type B $C\overline{1}$ and native C1 are also due to limited degradation during purification. Further studies are obviously required to provide an answer to this question.

Acknowledgments — We thank Maxine F. Smolowitz and Ariela Ben-Shoshan for loyal and competent technical assistance. Thanks are also due to Dr. E. L. Becker, Walter Reed Army Institute of Pathology, for a generous supply of p-nitrophenylethyl benzyl phosphonate. We further thank Dr. K. Amiraian, Division of Laboratories, New York State Department of Health, for the guinea pig serum he has furnished us.

REFERENCES

1. Nishioka K., *Immunochemistry* **3**, 501 (1966).
2. Hoffmann L. G., *Science* **159**, 322 (1968).
3. Hoffmann L. G., McKenzie A. T. and Mayer M. M., *Immunochemistry* **2**, 31 (1965).
4. Hoffmann L. G., *Immunochemistry* **6**, 309 (1969).
5. Rapp H. J. and Borsos T., *J. Immun.* **91**, 826 (1963).
6. Borsos T. and Rapp H. J., *J. Immun.* **91**, 851 (1963).
7. Mayer M. M. and Miller J. A., *Immunochemistry* **2**, 71 (1965).

8. Hoffmann L. G. and Meier P., *Immunochemistry* **4**, 419 (1967).
9. Becker E. L. and Austen K. F., *J. exp. Med.* **120**, 491 (1964).
10. Hoffmann L. G., *J. Chromatog.* **40**, 39 (1969).
11. Borsos T., Rapp H. J. and Cook C. T., *J. Immun.* **87**, 330 (1961).
12. Hoffmann L. G. and McGivern P. W., *J. Chromatog.* **40**, 53 (1969).
13. Borsos T. and Rapp H. J., *J. Immun.* **95**, 559 (1965).
14. Gigli I., Ruddy S. and Austen K. F., *J. Immun.* **100**, 1154 (1968).
15. Borsos T., Rapp H. J. and Walz U. L., *J. Immun.* **92**, 108 (1964).
16. Linscott W. D., *Immunochemistry* **5**, 311 (1968).
17. McEwen C. R., *Anal. Biochem.* **21**, 114 (1967).
18. Lepow I. H., Naff G. B., Todd E. W., Pensky J. and Hinz C. F. Jr., *J. exp. Med.* **117**, 983 (1963).
19. Nagaki K. and Stroud R. M., *J. Immun.* **102**, 421 (1969).
20. Sitomer G., Stroud R. M. and Mayer M. M., *Immunochemistry* **3**, 57 (1966).
21. Borsos T. and Rapp H. J., *J. Immun.* **94**, 510 (1965).
22. Colten H. R., Borsos T. and Rapp H. J., *J. Immun.* **100**, 808 (1968).
23. Tamura N. and Nelson R. A., Jr., *J. Immun.* **101**, 1333 (1968).
24. Lepow I. H., Ratnoff O. D., Rosen F. S. and Pillemer L., *Proc. Soc. exp. Biol. Med.* **92**, 32 (1956).
25. Weiss A., *Fedn. Proc.* **27**, 313 (1968).
26. Lepow I. H., Ratnoff O. D. and Levy L. R., *J. exp. Med.* **107**, 451 (1958).
27. Levine L., *Biochim. biophys. Acta* **18**, 283 (1955).
28. Becker E. L., *Nature, Lond.* **176**, 1073 (1955).

CHEMICAL STUDIES ON C1q; A MODULATOR OF IMMUNOGLOBULIN BIOLOGY

Kunio Yonemasu, Robert M. Stroud, William Niedermeier
and William T. Butler

Summary: Complete amino acid analyses of purified C1q from human serum indicate that this glycoprotein has an unusual composition for a serum protein, which includes hydroxyproline, hydroxylysine and high levels of glycine. A majority of the hydroxylysine residues are resistant to periodate oxidation; presumably they are protected by linkages to carbohydrate groups. In addition the total carbohydrate content is 7.7%, consisting primarily of glucose and galactose in equimolar amounts. Smaller quantities of sialic acid, fucose, mannose, galactosamine and glucosamine were also found. Thus, the data indicate that C1q has a structural similarity to collagen and collagen-like proteins.

Introduction: Activation of the complement system by certain subclasses of the immunoglobulins IgG and IgM depends on their interaction with a human serum protein designated C1q (1). C1q was first described by Müller-Eberhard and Kunkel (2), who noted precipitation when IgG and human serum were mixed. A protein (C1q) with an 11S sedimentation constant was recovered from this precipitate and shown to be important in the expression of the hemolytic activity of the complement system. In addition to immunoglobulin binding, C1q interacts with two other serum proteins, C1r and C1s, to form the first component of the human complement system, C1 (3). Therefore it is a physical link between certain immunoglobulins and one of their important effector systems.

Because of its ability to combine preferentially with altered immunoglobulins and certain polyanionic materials, this protein has been useful clinically to detect altered immunoglobulins, antigen-antibody complexes, and endotoxin (4). IgM immunoglobulins have been divided into two major classes on the basis of their ability to bind C1q (5). C1q may also be involved in IgG catabolism or synthesis (6,7). The results of our chemical analyses of C1q are given in this report. By use of a rapid and efficient purification method yielding 60%

116

recovery, we have been able to prepare Clq in sufficient quantity to permit determination of its amino acid composition, carbohydrate composition and the probable mode of attachment of at least some of the carbohydrate units. The results indicate that Clq has a chemical similarity to collagen and collagen-like proteins (e.g. basement membrane proteins).

Methods: Clq was purified with a 50-60% yield from whole human serum by using a method of repetitive precipitation in low ionic strength buffers containing chelating agents (8). The purity and homogeneity of these Clq preparations was shown immunochemically and electrophoretically. Only a single band could be demonstrated by immunoelectrophoresis against anti-serum to human serum and on polyacrylamide gel electrophoresis (Fig. 1). Also, immunoglobulins were not detected in these preparations of Clq using radial immunodiffusion. The limit of detection of IgG, IgM and IgA by this method is approximately 10, 5 and 15 µg/ml, respectively. These Clq preparations were tested at concentrations of Clq in excess of 1 mg/ml. Calculations based on these data indicate that immunoglobulin contamination could account for no more than 0.2 grams of carbohydrate per 100 grams of Clq.

The biological activity of these preparations was checked by the previously described methods (8). The characteristic hemolytic activity and latex agglutination activity was found, and there were no detectable Clr and Cls activities (8). Moreover, these preparations of Clq precipitated heat denatured IgG (1,4).

The molecular weight was found to be 388,000 (8) in agreement with a previous report (1). Nitrogen determination was done by sulfuric acid digestion followed by Nesslerization (9). Ammonium sulfate and crystalline human serum albumin were used as primary standards. As Clq is heat labile, drying to a constant weight after lyophilization was carried out at 40° C. Higher drying temperature caused denaturation and decreased the solubility. Amino acid analysis was performed on a single column automatic amino acid analyzer modified for high speed analysis (10). Samples were hydrolyzed for 24 hours in constant boiling HCl at 108° C under nitrogen.

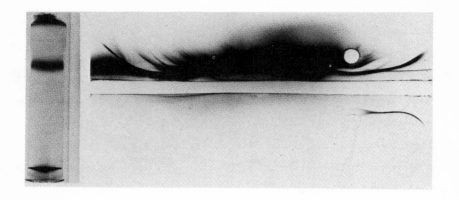

Figure 1. Purity of Clq. This preparation of Clq was purified from out-dated
serum by repeated precipitation as described (8).
A. Immunoelectrophoresis (anode is to the right). Upper well,
normal whole human serum: lower well, purified Clq: trough,
horse anti-whole human serum.
B. Acrylamide gel disc electrophoresis. The buffer contains 0.1%
sodium-dodecyl sulfate (S.D.S.), pH 8.3 (cathode is at the
top). The purified Clq sample contained 5% sucrose and 0.75%
S.D.S. The band near the anode is a non-specific band which
forms at the buffer interface.

The carbohydrate composition was determined on 3-5 mg portions of lyophil-

ized Clq dried to a constant weight at 40° C in vacuo. The carbohydrate analyses

employed a gas chromatographic method (11). When necessary, in order to comple-

tely solubilize Clq, pepsin was added at an enzyme to substrate ratio of 1:100

and reacted overnight at 37° C. After pepsin proteolysis, samples were hydro-

lyzed in 1N HCl at 100° C for 1, 4 and 10 hours. Arabinose and galactosamine

were added as internal standards for the neutral and amino sugars respectively.

The samples were reduced at 4° C with sodium borohydride and acetylated with

acetic anhydride in pyridine at 100° C. The alditol acetates were analysed

using glass columns packed with 1% ECNSS-M on 60/80 mesh Gas Chrom. Q (Applied

Science Laboratory, State College, Pennsylvania). Sialic acid determinations

were done by the thiobarbituric acid method of Warren (12). The amino sugars
were also assayed on the same columns used for amino acid analysis.

To determine the presence of hydroxylysine linked glycosides, the hydroxylysine content of a Clq preparation was compared before and after treatment
with periodate (13). The periodate was removed by dialysis before amino acid
analysis. Samples of rat skin collagen, which are known to contain periodate-
resistant hydroxylysine served as controls for this procedure.

Results:

Chemical Composition of Clq. The nitrogen content of Clq was found to be
13.2 ± 0.2%. The extinction coefficient in 1% sodium–dodecyl sulfate ($E_{1cm}^{1\%}$)
was found to be 6.8 ± 0.4 at 278 nm. Ultraviolet absorption spectra show a
single peak between 251 and 320 nm at 278 nm.

The amino acid composition of Clq, given in Table 1, is unusual for a
serum protein as it contains the amino acids 4-hydroxyproline and hydroxylysine

Table 1: Amino Acid Composition of Clq*

	Residues per Thousand	Residues per Mole
4-Hydroxyproline	38.9	130
Aspartic Acid	85.0	285
Threonine	52.7	177
Serine	55.2	185
Glutamic Acid	91.9	308
Proline	60.3	202
Glycine	173.2	580
Alanine	44.2	148
Cysteine†	24.6	82
Valine	55.2	185
Methionine	25.4	85
Isoleucine	38.1	128
Leucine	60.0	201
Tyrosine	30.2	101
Phenylalanine	42.4	142
Tryptophan††	9.1	30
Hydroxylysine	18.8	63
Lysine	36.8	123
Histidine	14.0	47
Arginine	42.9	144
Total		3346

*Values are the average of four separate analyses. No corrections were made
  for losses of serine, threonine, or tyrosine during hydrolysis.
†Determined as cysteic acid after performic acid oxidation (14).
††Determined spectrophotometrically (15).

and unusually high amounts of glycine and proline. A previous report mentions
the high glycine and hydroxylysine content, but the data were not complete (1).

The average carbohydrate content was determined on two separate Clq samples
prepared from different sera. The mean total carbohydrate content determined as
the sum of the monosaccharides was 7.7%. The monosaccharides found to be
present in Clq are shown in Table 2. Although the method of analysis would have
detected the presence of other monosaccharides, none were observed. Noteworthy
are the relatively high concentrations of glucose and galactose in a ratio of
1:1, and the presence of both glucosamine and galactosamine in a ratio of 2:1.

Table 2: Carbohydrate Composition of Clq

Carbohydrate	%	residues/mole MW = 388,000
Fucose	0.13	3.1
Mannose	0.87	18.6
Galactose	2.62	56.5
Glucose	2.53	54.5
Glucosamine*	0.92	20.0
Galactosamine*	0.43	9.4
Sialic acid†	0.31	2.9
Total	7.72	165

*Calculated as free base
†Calculated as N-acetylneuraminic acid

Carbohydrate Linkage to Hydroxylysine. Since the amino acid composition of Clq
exhibited a similarity to collagen and to the collagen-related proteins of basement membranes (16), it seemed possible that glucose and galactose were linked
to hydroxylysine. To test this possibility the degree of susceptibility of

Table 3: The Effect of Periodate on the Hydroxylysine Levels of Collagen and
Clq*

	Ratio Hydroxylysine:Phenylalanine		Hydroxylysine Remaining %
	Untreated	Treated	
Collagen	0.540	0.165	30
Clq	0.475	0.277	58

*Values are normalized by comparison of the levels of hydroxylysine to those
of phenylalanine, an amino acid unaffected by the periodate treatment. The
values are an average of two separate experiments.

120

hydroxylysine to periodate oxidation was determined. In Clq 58% of the hydroxy-lysine residues were protected from destruction by periodate (Table 3), suggest-ing that indeed, the hydroxyl groups of a number of the hydroxylysine side chains are substituted, most probably by glycosides.

Discussion: This serum protein contains relatively more hydroxylysine but some-what less hydroxyproline and glycine than most collagens. The overall composi-tion is more reminiscent of basement membrane proteins than of collagen (17), and portions of Clq may be homologous to the α chains of collagen. The large amount of carbohydrate in Clq (Table 2) and the large percentage of hydroxy-lysine residues which are apparently glycosylated (Table 3) also suggest a closer relationship of Clq to basement membranes than to collagen. It is interesting to note, however, that Clq does not contain 3-hydroxyproline, where-as this isomer constitutes a substantial proportion of the hydroxyproline of basement membranes (17).

The failure of 58% of the hydroxylysine residues to undergo periodate oxidation together with the observation that glucose and galactose are present in relatively large, equimolar quantities, suggests that Clq may contain gluco-sylgalactosyl-hydroxylysine units similar to those reported for basement membranes (18), collagens (13,19) and the lens capsule (20). The other sugars present presumably represent heteropolysaccharide units analogous to those found associated with the renal glomerular basement membranes (21). It is also known that Clq with a molecular weight of approximately 388,000, has an inter-esting subunit (8) and electron microscopic structure (22). It is electropho-retically one of the slowest moving proteins in human serum at pH 8.6 and the least soluble at low ionic strength (8). Further chemical studies on this important and unique serum protein are in progress. Delineation of the binding sites on Clq for IgG and IgM will facilitate our understanding of the biolog-ical effects of these immunoglobulin subclasses.

Acknowledgement: We acknowledge many helpful discussions with Dr. J. C. Bennett and the technical assistance of Miss Freda Moore.

121

This research was supported by grants from the N.I.H. and Veterans Administration and Grant No. DE - 02670 from the N.I.D.R.

References

1. Müller-Eberhard, H. J., Ann. Rev. Biochem., 38, 389 (1969).
2. Müller-Eberhard, H. J. and H. G. Kunkel, Proc. Soc. Exp. Biol. Med., 106, 291 (1960).
3. Lepow, I. H., G. B. Naff, W. D. Todd, J. Pensky and C. F. Hinz, J. Exp. Med., 117, 983 (1963).
4. Agnello, V., R. J. Winchester and H. G. Kunkel, Immunology, 19, 909 (1970).
5. Linscott, W. D. and S. S. Hansen, J. Immunol., 103, 423 (1969).
6. Kohler, P. F. and H. J. Müller-Eberhard, Science, 163, 474 (1969).
7. Stroud, R. M., K. Nagaki, R. J. Pickering, H. Gewurz, R. A. Good and M. D. Cooper, Clin. and Exptl. Immunology, 7, 133 (1970).
8. Yonemasu, K. and R. M. Stroud, J. Immunol., 106, 304 (1971).
9. Chase, M. W. and C. A. Williams, in Methods in Immunology and Immunochemistry, Vol. II, 266-270, Academic Press, 1968.
10. Miller, E. J. and K. A. Piez, Anal. Biochem., 16, 320 (1966).
11. Niedermeier, W., Anal. Biochem., (accepted, to be published 1971).
12. Warren, L., J. Biol. Chem., 234, 1971 (1959).
13. Butler, W. T. and L. W. Cunningham, J. Biol. Chem., 241, 3882 (1966).
14. Moore, S., J. Biol. Chem., 238, 235 (1963).
15. Spande, T. F. and B. Witkop, in Methods in Enzymology, Vol. XI, 498, Academic Press, 1967.
16. Spiro, R. G. in Chemistry and Molecular Biology of the Intercellular Matrix, Vol. I, 511, Academic Press, 1970.
17. Kefalides, N. A. in Chemistry and Molecular Biology of the Intercellular Matrix, Vol. I, 535, Academic Press, 1970.
18. Spiro, R. G., J. Biol. Chem., 244, 602 (1969).
19. Spiro, R. G., J. Biol. Chem., 242, 4813 (1967).
20. Spiro, R. G. and Fukushi, S., J. Biol. Chem., 244, 2049 (1969).
21. Spiro, R. G., J. Biol. Chem., 242, 1923 (1967).
22. Shelton, E., K. Yonemasu and R. M. Stroud, J. Immunol., to be published 1971. Presented at the Fourth Complement Workshop, Baltimore, 1971. The abstracts of this meeting will be published in J. Immunol. 1971.

122

STRUCTURAL STUDIES ON HUMAN C1q: NON-COVALENT AND COVALENT SUBUNITS*†

KUNIO YONEMASU and ROBERT M. STROUD

Abstract — Highly purified C1q was dissociated into two subunits by urea and iodoacetamide. The molecular weight of these subunits was estimated by acrylamide gel containing SDS and was found to be 60,000 (I) and 42,000 (II). Furthermore after extensive reduction and alkylation of C1q, three subunits were found. The estimated molecular weight of these subunits was found to be 29,000 (I-1), 27,000 (I-2) and 22,000 (II-3) respectively. Moreover, it was found that the larger non-covalent subunit (I) dissociated upon reduction and alkylation into two of the smaller subunits, I-1 and I-2, and that the smaller non-covalent subunit (II) dissociated into the subunit, II-3. The molar ratios of the non-covalent and disulfide linked subunits were obtained by scanning acrylamide gels stained with Amido black. From the relative density of the protein bands and the estimated molecular weights, it was found that the relative molar ratios of I to II to the nearest integer was 3:1, and the molar ratios of the smaller subunits obtained after reduction and alkylation was 3:3:2 for I-1, I-2 and II-3 respectively. Therefore, in the intact molecule, we have postulated that human C1q consists of eight non-covalent subunits (six of I and two of II) and contains a total of sixteen smaller subunits (six of I-1, six of I-2 and four of II-3), pairs of which are held together by disulfide bonds.

By immunodiffusion it was shown that all of these subunits have a distinct antigenicity and that the antigenic determinants of intact C1q are lost upon reduction and alkylation. Antiserum to the reduced and alkylated polypeptide chains was produced in rabbits. This antiserum reacted with the non-covalent subunits as would be expected since they consist of pairs of the smaller disulfide linked subunits. The antigenicity of intact C1q was heat labile in contradistinction to the antigenicity of the non-covalent and covalent subunits.

INTRODUCTION

Human C1q was originally isolated by Müller-Eberhard and Kunkel (1961) who characterized this molecule as a heat labile 11S serum protein which was capable of interacting and precipitating soluble gamma globulin aggregates in the presence of EDTA. Lepow *et al.* (1963) separated three sub-components, C1q, C1r and C1s, from macromolecular C1 on DEAE cellulose in the presence of EDTA. They showed that these subunits could be recombined into hemolytic-

*Presented in part at the First International Congress of Immunology, Washington, D.C., August, 1971.

†Requests for reprints should be addressed to Dr. R. M. Stroud, Division of Clinical Immunology and Rheumatology, 1919 Seventh Avenue South, Birmingham, Alabama 35233, U.S.A.

ally active Cl by the addition of calcium. As Cl is known to combine with antigen–antibody complexes or aggregated immunoglobulins, and as Clq has an affinity for certain immunoglobulins, the immunoglobulin binding site of Cl is considered to be on the Clq sub-component of this macromolecule. The valency of Clq for IgG was reported by Müller-Eberhard (1969) to be approximately 5 as determined by ultracentrifugal analysis of Clq and IgG mixtures. The molecular weight of Clq has been reported to be 400,000 by Müller-Eberhard (1968) (sedimentation velocity) and 388,000 (acrylamide gel) in our previous report (Yonemasu and Stroud, 1971). In a recent study of the ultrastructure of Clq, Shelton *et al.* (1972), showed that the molecular consisted of six terminal subunits linked by connecting strands to a central subunit and that its overall diameter of approximately 350 Å was comparable to that of IgM (Chesebro *et al.*, 1968). Previous reports on the biochemical structure of Clq are not fully published, but Müller-Eberhard (1968) has found that urea starch gel electrophoresis of reduced and alkylated Clq reveals two subunits, one of which has a mobility similar to L chains from IgG.

Using the efficient purification method described previously (Yonemasu and Stroud, 1971) we have been able to prepare Clq in sufficient quantity to permit detailed studies of the polypeptide structure of Clq. Using this method of preparation the complete amino acid and carbohydrate composition of Clq was recently published (Yonemasu *et al.*, 1971). Both covalent and non-covalent subunits have been found, and from the estimates of the amount of each subunit the intact structure of Clq is hypothesized.

MATERIALS AND METHODS

(1) *Reagents*

Urea' was purchased from the J. T. Baker Chemical Co., Phillipsburg, N.J. Aqueous solutions of urea were absorbed repeatedly with activated charcoal until the absorbance at 280 nm was negligible. Iodoacetamide and dithiothreitol were purchased from Sigma Chemical Co., St. Louis, Missouri and Calbiochem, Los Angeles, California, respectively. Sodium dodecyl sulfate (SDS) was purchased from K & K Laboratories, Inc., Plainview, N.Y. Agarose was purchased from Bausch & Lomb Optical Co., Rochester, N.Y. Acrylamide (for electrophoresis) and N,N'-Methylenebisacrylamide were purchased from Eastman Kodak Co., Rochester, N.Y. Human IgG (fraction II) was a gift from Merck Sharp & Dohme Research Laboratories, West Point, Pa. Sulfitolyzed human IgG was kindly supplied by Dr. J. C. Bennett. Cytochrome c from horse heart, type III, was purchased from Sigma Chemical Co., St. Louis, Missouri. Horse antiserum to whole human serum was obtained from Microbiol Diseases Research Foundation, Osaka University, Osaka, Japan. Antisera to Clq were prepared as described (Yonemasu and Stroud, 1971).

(2) *Purification of human Clq*

Human Clq was purified from fresh or outdated human serum by repeated precipitation in EGTA and EDTA solutions as previously described (Yonemasu and Stroud, 1971). Since IgG and IgM contamination was occasionally found when outdated blood was used, an empirical modification of this method grad-

124

ually evolved. We used a slightly higher molarity of EGTA, $0.03\,M$, ($RSC^* = 0.035$, pH 7·5) for the first dialysis step. $0.069\,M$ EDTA ($RSC = 0.078$, pH 5·0) was used for the second dialysis step and $0.04\,M$ EDTA ($RSC = 0.075$, pH 7·5) for the final dialysis step. These conditions were found to simultaneously maximize Clq precipitation and minimize IgG, IgM and IgA contamination. It is necessary that the conditions be precisely controlled and pilot experiments may be necessary to determine the precise conditions. The dialysis times and the volume of fluid that is used for redissolving after each precipitation should be controlled as outlined previously (Yonemasu and Stroud, 1971). These Clq preparations were highly purified as shown by immunoelectrophoresis and analytical acrylamide gel electrophoresis (Fig. 1). Furthermore, immunoglobulins could not be detected in these preparations of Clq using radial immunodiffusion methods capable of detecting 10, 5 and 15 μg/ml of IgG, IgM and IgA respectively. Preparations of Clq were tested for purity at concentrations of approximately 1 mg/ml. Concentrations of Clq were determined by radial immunodiffusion as described (Yonemasu and Stroud, 1971) or spectrophotometrically when highly homogeneous, using the experimentally determined extinction coefficient of 6·8 at 278 nm (Yonemasu *et al.*, 1971). The biological activities of these Clq preparations were determined by the previously described methods (Yonemasu and Stroud, 1971), and hemolytic activity, precipitability of soluble aggregated IgG, and agglutination of IgG coated latex particles were intact. There was no detectable Clr and Cls activity.

(3) *Non-covalent subunits of* Clq

Purified Clq preparations at concentrations of 0·5–1 mg/ml were dialyzed against 8 M urea containing $0.01\,M$ iodoacetamide in $0.05\,M$ Tris buffer at pH 8·0 for approximately 16 hr at 2–4°C.

(4) *Reduction and alkylation of* Clq

Preparations of Clq at 0·5–1 mg/ml were incubated in $0.1\,M$ dithiothreitol containing 8 M urea and $0.1\,M$ Tris buffer at pH 8·0 for 4 hr at room temperature. Alkylation was carried out with a 2-fold molar excess of iodoacetamide at pH 8·0 for 15 min at room temperature. The pH during the alkylation was maintained by the addition of 1 M Tris.

(5) *Antiserum to the reduced and alkylated subunits of* Clq

Purified Clq was obtained by precipitating normal human serum first in EGTA ($RSC = 0.035$, pH 7·5 at 2–4°C, overnight) then in EDTA ($RSC = 0.078$, pH 5·0 at 2–4°C for 4 hr). This was followed by two identical preparative acrylamide gel electrophoresis runs using the previously described gel electrophoresis conditions at pH 8·3 in 0·1% SDS (Yonemasu and Stroud, 1971). The gel segments containing Clq were pulverized and then reduced and alkylated, using the

*The RSC (relative salt concentration) of a solution is the concentration of a NaCl solution which gives the same electrical resistance at 0°C. This is determined from a previously prepared standard graph. The EDTA and EGTA solutions do not contain any other salts except for the NaOH used for adjustment of pH. If necessary, distilled water is used to give a final adjustment of the RSC.

conditions described above. After reduction and alkylation, preparations were dialyzed against $0.15\,M$ NaCl and then mixed with equal volumes of Freund's complete adjuvant. Each rabbit was immunized intradermally or subcutaneously with approximately 200 μg of protein at intervals of 3–4 weeks for several months until precipitating antiserum was obtained.

(6) Acrylamide gel disc electrophoresis

In order to check the purity of Clq on acrylamide gel disc electrophoresis a modification of the method of Davis (1964) was used. The gel and electrode buffer contained 0.1% SDS at pH 8·3. Usually 0.05 ml of the sample, containing 0.75% SDS and 10% sucrose was applied to the top of the gel (running gel, measured 0.5×4.0 cm, and concentrating gel 0.5×1.0 cm). For electrophoresis of the subunits, gels containing $0.5\,M$ urea and 0.1% SDS as described by Williamson and Askonas (1968), were used at pH 7·2. Generally, 0.05 ml of the sample, containing $1\,M$ urea and 0.75% SDS, was applied on the top of gel columns measuring 0.6×7.0 cm.

(7) Immunodiffusion analysis

(a) Ouchterlony double diffusion was carried out using 1% agarose dissolved in $0.05\,M$ Tris and $0.05\,M$ glycine-buffered saline ($0.15\,M$ NaCl). One M urea was also added to maintain the solubility of Clq. The final RSC was 0.185 at pH 8·0. (b) Immunoelectrophoresis of Clq was carried out according to a modification of the method of Scheidegger (1955) using 1% agarose in veronal acetate buffer containing $0.01\,M$ EDTA. Analysis of the subunits of Clq was carried out on 1% agarose dissolved in $0.05\,M$ Tris and $0.05\,M$ glycine-buffered saline ($0.15\,M$ NaCl) containing $1\,M$ urea (RSC = 0.183, pH 8·6). The electrode buffer was the same except that it contained $0.5\,M$ urea instead of $1\,M$ urea.

(8) Molecular weight estimation of the subunits of Clq

The molecular weights were estimated according to a modification of the method of Dunker and Rueckert (1969), using acrylamide gels (measuring 0.6×7.0 cm) containing $0.5\,M$ urea and 0.1% SDS at pH 7·2. Various concentrations of polyacrylamide gels were used as noted. Human IgG (160,000) μ-chains (75,000) from sulfitolyzed human IgM, and reduced and alkylated human IgG (γ-chain, 55,000; L-chain, 22,500) (Edelman and Marchalonis, 1968) were used as markers with known molecular weights. Cytochrome c was used as a reference point for the relative mobilities of the other proteins.

(9) Molar ratios of Clq subunits

Acrylamide gels were stained with Amido black according to Parish and Marchalonis (1970) and scanned using a Gilford Densitometer, Model 2000, Gilford Instrument Laboratories, Inc., Oberlin, Ohio. The areas below the curves were determined by planimetry, and the molar ratios calculated from the molecular weights of the subunits.

RESULTS

(1) Subunits of Clq

The non-covalent linkage of certain Clq subunits was suspected when the breakdown of intact Clq was noted on gels containing sodium dodecyl sulfate in the presence of $0.5\,M$ urea. However, there was a high proportion of intact molecules and higher molecular weight aggregates. Consequently, Clq was deliberately incubated with $8\,M$ urea containing $0.01\,M$ iodoacetamide to prevent disulfide interchange. This treatment completely dissociated Clq (see methods section) into two distinct protein bands as shown in Fig. 2 (1). We have designated these two non-covalent subunits I and II in order of their relative molecular weights. On most of these gels there is a small amount of higher molecular weight materials (3–9 per cent by scanning) usually distributed in two bands. These bands have a calculated molecular weight corresponding to dimers of each of these subunits. Also, in Fig. 2 (2) this gel shows reduced and alkylated Clq using the identical gel electrophoresis conditions. Reducing conditions were studied in order to determine empirically the conditions which yield a complete breakdown of intact Clq as determined by inspection of the acrylamide gels. As shown, reduction in $0.1\,M$ dithiothreitol containing $8\,M$ urea followed by alkylation gives protein bands which we have designated I-1, I-2, and II-3 in order of their molecular weights. The nomenclature of the various Clq subunits is summarized in Table 1. Reduction in $0.1\,M$ dithiothreitol without urea produced subunits with molecular weights of 150,000 and 220,000, although higher polymers were also obtained, suggesting a varying susceptibility to reduction of the disulfide bonds of Clq.

Table 1. Summary of the subunit structure of human Clq. Note each I probably consists of I-1 and I-2. Each II consists of two II-3

Designation of Subunit	Type of Binding	Estimated mol. wt.	Proposed Number in Intact Clq
I	Non covalent	60,000	6
II	Non covalent	42,000	2
I-1	Covalent	29,000	6
I-2	Covalent	27,000	6
II-3	Covalent	22,000	4

(2) *Immunodiffusion analysis of* Clq *and its subunits*

The non-covalent subunits of Clq prepared as above by incubation in $8\,M$ urea and $0.01\,M$ iodoacetamide, and the subunits of Clq obtained after complete reduction and alkylation were compared on immunoelectrophoresis at pH 8.6 to the highly purified preparation of Clq from which they were obtained. As shown in Fig. 3, antiserum to Clq showed a single precipitation line against purified Clq and the mobility of Clq was characteristically found to be in the slow gamma region. The mobility of the three subunits was found to be in the gamma to beta globulin region. Antisera to intact Clq did not react with the subunits in these experiments. The antiserum used to detect these was prepared by immunization with the reduced and alkylated subunits as detailed above. Although the three subunits could not be separated distinctly under these conditions, the electrophoretic pattern is slightly different from the parent molecule. On Ouchterlony double diffusion (Fig. 4) the antiserum to the intact molecule showed only a

127

faint reaction with the reduced and alkylated subunits. The antiserum to the reduced and alkylated subunits did not show any detectable precipitation with the intact molecule but did show two precipitation arcs with the non-covalent subunits. Three distinct precipitate arcs were apparent with this antisera and a reduced and alkylated Clq preparation. These three arcs presumably correspond to the three subunits visualized on acrylamide gel electrophoresis (Fig. 2 (2)). Two of these reduced and alkylated subunit arcs appeared to fuse with one of the non-covalent subunit bands and the third reduced and alkylated arc fused with the other non-covalent subunit arc, suggesting that one of the urea subunits is made up of two of the reduced and alkylated subunits. This relationship was determined more definitively on acrylamide gel electrophoresis as discussed below. Also the heat lability of the antigenic determinants of the intact Clq molecule, relative to its subunits, is shown in Fig. 4. Clq and the various types of subunit mixtures were incubated individually at 56°C for 90 min. Note that Clq loses most of its capacity to precipitate with these antisera. However, the determinants on the subunits of Clq apparently were not affected by heating at the same temperature. These experiments suggest that intact Clq has antigenic determinants which are primarily determined by the conformation of the molecule in spite of its lability. However, the antigenic determinants of the covalent and non-covalent subunits are less dependent on a labile conformational structure and are distinct from those on the intact structure.

(3) *Estimation of the molecular weight of the non-covalent and covalent subunits of* Clq

The molecular weights of all the subunits were estimated by their relative mobility on acrylamide gel electrophoresis in relationship to the molecular weights of known proteins and polypeptide chains. Polyacrylamide gels at concentrations of 5% and 7% gave a linear relationship when the logarithm of the molecular weight was graphed as a function of the relative migration distance (Fig. 5). The molecular weights of subunits I, II, I-1, I-2 and II-3 were found to be approximately 60,000, 42,000, 29,000, 27,000 and 22,000 respectively (summarized in Table 1). It was of interest that if protein markers, which were not single randomly oriented polypeptide chains, were used, the values were slightly higher, as was noted previously (Yonemasu and Stroud, 1971). The lower values are presumably more correct due to the random coil of the markers (Fish *et al.*, 1970).

(4) *Relationship of the non-covalent subunits* (I *and* II) *to the covalent subunits* (I-1, I-2 *and* II-3)

The mixture of subunits obtained after urea and iodoacetamide incubation at a concentration of 4 mg/ml was subjected to preparative acrylamide gel electrophoresis (8% gel, 1.15×7.0 cm) containing $0.5\,M$ urea and 0.1% SDS at pH 7.2. Subunits I and II were eluted from the gel segments with small volumes of $8\,M$ urea in $0.05\,M$ Tris buffer at pH 8.0, after examination of a stained longitudinally cut strip of the gel to locate them. The eluates containing I and II were then individually reduced and alkylated. As shown in Fig. 6, reduction and alkylation of II yielded a single protein band with a mobility corresponding to the smallest subunit (II-3), obtained after reduction and alkylation of intact Clq.

128

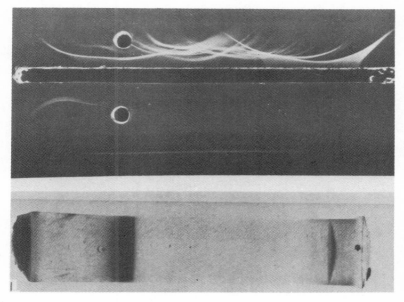

Fig. 1. Purity of Clq.

An immunoelectrophoresis of a Clq preparation prepared from outdated sera by repeated precipitation in low molarities of EGTA and EDTA is shown. The antiserum is an antiserum to whole human serum. The lower picture shows the stained acrylamide gel for this preparation. The anode is to the right. The applied sample was highly purified Clq at a concentration of 430 μg/ml. The gel was 4% acrylamide and the buffer contained 0·1% SDS, pH 8·3. The Clq sample was in 0·75% SDS and 10% sucrose. The band near the anode is a non-specific band which forms at the water–buffer interface.

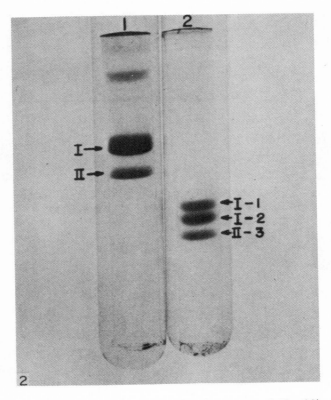

Fig. 2. Acrylamide gel electrophoresis of the subunits of Clq. 8% gels containing $0.5\,M$ urea and 0.1% SDS at pH 7.2 were used. The cathode is at the top and the gels were stained with Amido black.

(1) Non-covalent subunits of Clq.

Clq was treated with urea and iodoacetamide (see text) and was applied to the top of a gel. Note that two subunits are seen and designated I and II in order of their molecular weights.

(2) Covalent subunits of Clq.

Clq was fully reduced and alkylated at a concentration of 780 μg/ml. The three protein bands, designated I-1, I-2 and II-3, in order of their molecular weights are noted.

130

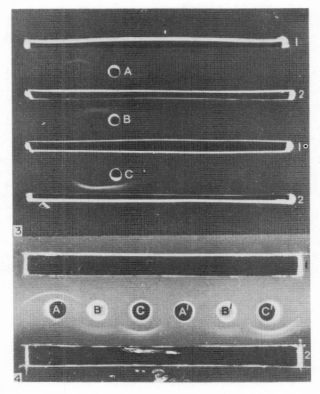

Fig. 3. Immunodiffusion analysis of Clq and its subunits.

Immunoelectrophoresis (the anode is to the right). Well *A* contains purified Clq. Well *B* contains the non-covalent subunits after 8 *M* urea and 0·01 *M*
iodoacetamide treatment and well *C* contains reduced and alkylated subunits.
These subunits are prepared from the identical Clq preparation in well *A*.
Trough 1 contains antiserum to Clq and 2 contains antiserum to reduced and
alkylated subunits.

Fig. 4. Ouchterlony diffusion.

Wells *A*, *B* and *C* and troughs 1 and 2 contain the identical samples used
for the above mentioned immunoelectrophoresis (see Fig. 3). Wells *A'*, *B'* and
C' contain the same samples after incubating them at 56°C for 90 mins. Although it is difficult to see there are three bands between well *C* and well *C'*
and trough 2 and the third band fuses incompletely with one of the urea
subunits.

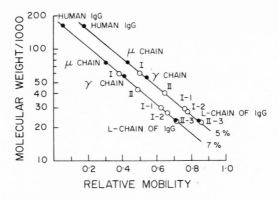

Fig. 5. Molecular weight of subunits.
This graph shows the logarithm of the molecular weights of reference proteins in relation to their relative mobilities on 5% and 7% polyacrylamide gels containing 0·5 M urea and 0·1% SDS at pH 7·2. The reference proteins were run on the same gel and cytochrome c was used as a reference point.
The positions of the subunits I, II, I-1, I-2 and II-3 are shown.

Reduction and alkylation of I yielded two protein bands with mobilities corresponding exactly to I-1 and I-2 which were obtained after reduction and alkylation of intact Clq. These relationships are compatible with the molecular weights of I, II, I-1, I-2 and II-3 found in the preceeding experiment. Division of the molecular weight of II by 2 is approximately equal to the molecular weight of II-3. The molecular weight of I is equal to the sum of the molecular weight of I-1 plus the molecular weight of I-2, within the experimental error of the methods.

(5) *Relative proportions of the subunits of* Clq

Intact acrylamide gels from the previously described experiments (result section 4) were stained with Amido black and scanned using a Gilford Densitometer. Figure 7(1) shows an actual scan of a single experiment; a total of three experiments were done. In this experiment the relative areas under the density curves of I and II were found to be 77 per cent and 17 per cent, respectively. Six per cent of the protein was accounted for in a higher molecular weight band which on elution and repeat electrophoresis was found to dissociate into I and/or II. From the estimated molecular weights, the calculated molar ratio of these subunits was found to be 3·28:1·00. The average of three experiments was found to be 2·89:1·00, which was rounded off to 3:1 in order to build a molecular model.

Similarly, gel scanning of the completely reduced and alkylated subunits shows that the relative protein amounts of I-1, I-2 and II-3 were found to be 39 per cent, 40 per cent and 21 per cent. Calculated molar ratios were therefore 2·80:3·14:2·00 respectively. These data are shown in Fig. 7 (2). The three experiments agreed well and were averaged. The averages were 39 per cent, 39 per cent and 22 per cent. Therefore the average calculated molar ratios were 2·76:

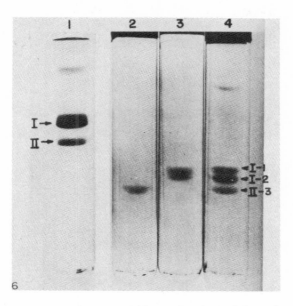

Fig. 6. Relation between the non-covalent subunits and the reduced and alkylated subunits.

Acrylamide gels (8% gels) containing 0·5 M urea, 0·1% SDS, pH 7·2 were run (cathode is at the top). The gels were stained with Coomassie blue.

Gel 1: The applied sample was the mixture of non-covalent subunits of Clq obtained after 8 M urea and 0·01 M iodoacetamide.

Gel 2: To the top of this gel was applied the reduced and alkylated eluate containing the smaller non-covalent subunit (II) with a molecular weight of 42,000. Only a single subunit is obtained with a mobility corresponding to II-3.

Gel 3: The larger non-covalent subunit (I) was eluted and reduced and alkylated. It was then applied to the top of this gel. Note that two polypeptide chains at the mobilities corresponding to I-1 and I-2 were obtained.

Gel 4: This gel contains the subunits of Clq obtained after extensive reduction and alkylation of intact Clq. Note that three distinct subunits (designated I-1, I-2 and II-3) are obtained.

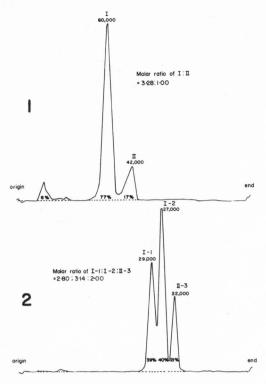

Fig. 7. Relative proportions of the Clq subunits by gel scanning.

This graph is an actual representation of a gel scan using a Gilford Densitometer. Gels were stained with Amido black.

Graph 1: Represents the subunits of Clq obtained after treatment with urea and 0·01 M iodoacetamide only so these are the non-covalent subunits designated I and II.

Graph 2: The subunits of Clq after extensive reduction and alkylation. These are the subunits designated I-1, I-2 and II-3. The origin and the end of each gel, the relative protein concentrations and the molecular weights are marked in the figure as are their calculated molar ratios. The areas were obtained from these curves by planimetry.

2·94:2·00. It should be noted that these molar ratios are consistent with I, dissociating into I-1 and I-2 as shown in the previous experiment. The ratios are also consistent with a mole of II dissociating into two moles of II-3. The nomenclature of the subunits was chosen to reflect these relationships and it has been summarized in Table 1.

DISCUSSION

Clq is an important serum glycoprotein as it directly combines with immunoglobulins and other proteins in the complement system and is therefore a link between immunoglobulins and the activation of the complement system. These studies have delineated the polypeptide structure of Clq and found it to consist of both covalently and non-covalently linked subunits. Treatment of human Clq with 8 M urea and 0·01 M iodoacetamide resulted in two distinct protein bands which we have designated I and II (see Table 1). Moreover, total reduction of Clq by 0·1 M dithiothreitol followed by alkylation resulted in three distinct protein bands designated I-1, I-2 and II-3. The estimated molecular weights of these subunits, I, II, I-1, I-2 and II-3, were found to be 60,000, 42,000, 29,000, 27,000 and 22,000, respectively. It was also noted that subunit I yielded the subunits I-1 and I-2 and that the subunit II yielded the subunits II-3 on reduction and alkylation. The gel scanning data suggested that the non-covalent subunits of Clq; i.e. those which dissociated in urea, had a molar ratio of 3 : 1 in favor of the larger subunit (I). Therefore, if one Clq molecule with an approximate molecular weight of 400,000 was composed of three of the 60,000 molecular weight subunits and one of the 42,000 molecular weight subunit, the total molecular weight would only be 222,000. However, if the molar ratio is multiplied by 2 and the molecular weight of the subunits are added, a molecular weight of approximately 444,000 is obtained. This would be within the experimental error of the gel scanning and the molecular weight estimation methods. Therefore, using these data Clq most likely has eight non-covalently linked subunits. Of these non-covalent subunits, six are made up of the two larger reduced and alkylated subunits (I-1 and I-2), and the other two are each dimers of the two smaller reduced and alkylated subunits (II-3). This model preserves the molar ratios of three independent experiments and is a reasonable hypothesis. As the non-covalent subunits contain disulfide bonds it is probable that their molecular weights are somewhat in error (Fish *et al.*, 1970). In our experiments employing unreduced proteins as markers, molecular weights which were approximately 10–15 per cent higher were found. Consequently, this error may not be significant. It is possible that we have overlooked subunits which are small and have too low a molar ratio to be found on acrylamide gels; however, staining with the sensitive Coomassie blue method did not suggest this.

Clq was recently shown (Shelton *et al.*, 1972) to be made up of six terminal subunits linked by connecting strands to a central subunit, and evidence was presented that the terminal and central parts of the molecule were each divided into two smaller components. These findings are compatible with the chemical data. Thus, the non-covalent subunit, I, could be equated with the terminal subunits and connecting strands, while the covalent subunits, I-1 and I-2, could be equated with the smaller components of the terminal subunits which appeared in the electron micrographs to be of unequal size and to have the connecting strands attached to the larger of the two. The central part of the molecule and its two apparently equal divisions may be equivalent to the two identical non-covalent subunits, II, which are each dimers of II-3. Currently this is our working hypothesis to correlate the chemical and microscopic data.

All of the reduced and alkylated polypeptide chains have antigenic determinants which appear to differ from the intact molecule but not from the non-covalent subunits. The non-covalent subunits are antigenically related to the covalently linked subunits as would be expected from the relationships that were found by acrylamide gel electrophoresis. The intact Clq molecule has antigenic determinants which are readily lost after heating, reduction and alkylation or urea treatment. This would indicate that Clq has a labile conformational structure dependent upon interacting subunits. It is well known that the biological function of Clq is also heat labile (Müller-Eberhard and Kunkel, 1961).

Obviously it is important to relate this subunit structure to the function of Clq. As Clq is known to combine with immunoglobulins and with Clr and Cls, and as the valence for immunoglobulins is approximately 5 or 6, (Müller-Eberhard, 1969), it is possible that the six subunits (I) have binding sites for immunoglobulins and that the subunits (II) moderate the binding of Clr and Cls. Again, this is a simple working hypothesis and will require further verification.

Acknowledgement — This research was supported by grants from the NIH and the Veterans Administration.

REFERENCES

Chesbro B., Bloth B. and Svehag S. E. (1968) *J. exp. Med.* **127**, 399.
Davis B. J. (1964) *Ann. N.Y. Acad. Sci.* **121**, 304.
Dunker A. K. and Rueckert R. R. (1969) *J. biol. Chem.* **244**, 5074.
Edelman G. M. and Marchalonis J. J. (1968) *Methods in Immunology and Immunochemistry*, Vol. I, chapter 5, p. 405. Academic Press, New York and London.
Fish W. W., Reynolds J. A. and Tanford C. (1970) *J. biol. Chem.* **245**, 5166.
Lepow I. H., Naff G. B., Todd W. D., Pensky J. and Hinz C. F. (1963) *J. exp. Med.* **117**, 983.
Müller-Eberhard H. J. (1968) *Adv. Immunol.* **8**, 1.
Müller-Eberhard H. J. (1969) *Ann. Rev. Biochem.* **38**, 389.
Müller-Eberhard H. J. and Kunkel H. G. (1961) *Proc. Soc. exp. Biol. Med.* **106**, 291.
Parish C. R. and Marchalonis J. J. (1970) *Analyt. Biochem.* **34**, 436.
Scheidegger J. J. (1955) *Int. Archs Allergy* **7**, 103.
Shelton E., Yonemasu K. and Stroud R. M. (1971) *J. Immun.* **107**, 310.
Shelton E., Yonemasu K. and Stroud R. M. (1972) *Proc. natn Acad. Sci. U.S.A.* **69**, 65.
Williamson A. R. and Askonas B. A. (1968) *Biochem. J.* **107**, 823.
Yonemasu K. and Stroud R. M. (1971) *J. Immun.* **106**, 304.
Yonemasu K. and Stroud R. M. (1971) *J. Immun.* **107**, 309.
Yonemasu K., Stroud R. M., Niedermeier W. and Butler W. T. (1971) *Biochem. biophys. Res. Commun.* **43**, 1388.

Ultrastructure of the Human Complement Component, Clq

Emma Shelton, Kunio Yonemasu, and Robert M. Stroud

ABSTRACT   The human complement component, Clq, is a fragile molecule of delicate structure consisting of three distinct parts, a central subunit, connecting strands, and terminal subunits. Each terminal subunit is further subdivided into a large and a small subunit, and the central subunit appears to be divided into two equal parts. In the intact molecule, six connecting strands link six terminal subunits by their larger subdivision to the central subunit. The overall diameter of the molecule when viewed from the "top" is about 35 nm (350 Å).

The human serum protein, Clq, binds specifically to certain subclasses of the immunoglobulins IgG and IgM and initiates the cascade of complex interactions that occurs among complement proteins (1). Since the molecule occupies a strategic position as the physical link between complement proteins and antigen–antibody complexes, knowledge of its ultrastructure may provide clues as to how it functions in this role.

Some indication of the possible structure of the molecule is supplied by physico-chemical data. Clq has a sedimentation coefficient of 11.1 and a molecular weight of about 400,000. It is a glycoprotein of unusual composition (1–4); the presence of hydroxyproline, hydroxylysine, and high levels of glycine in Clq indicate that it has a chemical structure similar to collagen-like proteins (4). There is substantial evidence that the molecule is made up of both covalently and noncovalently linked subunits (2, 3; Yonemasu and Stroud, submitted for

Abbreviations: EGTA, ethyleneglycol bis(aminoethyl)-tetraacetic acid; RSC, relative salt concentration.

publication) and a recent study of the ultrastructure of Clq has emphasized its extreme lability (5). We find the intact Clq molecule to consist of six terminal subunits joined by tenuous connections to a large central subunit.

METHODS

Preparation of Clq. Clq was prepared according to the method of Yonemasu and Stroud (3), which was modified slightly in order to provide molecules in a high state of purity. The electron micrographs illustrating this paper were derived from two experiments in which the purity of the samples was tested and in which both active and inactive Clq molecules were examined.

About 200 ml of freshly drawn blood from a male donor was allowed to clot at room temperature for 90 min. The serum was separated from the clot by a preliminary centrifugation at 500 × g for 20 min, followed by a second centrifugation at 900 × g for 20 min. The separated serum (63 ml) was then centrifuged at 41,300 × g for 90 min for the removal of free lipid and insoluble aggregates. The clear supernatant (57 ml) was dialyzed in the cold with stirring against 1 liter of 0.03 M ethyleneglycol bis(aminoethyl)-tetraacetic acid (EGTA), relative salt concentration (RSC) 0.036, pH 7.5 (ref. 3; Yonemasu and Stroud, submitted for publication) for 4.5 hr and then overnight against 1 liter of fresh EGTA. The resulting precipitate was centrifuged and washed twice with 0.03 M EGTA (pH 7.5, RSC 0.036). The washed precipitate was redissolved to 11 ml with 0.75 M NaCl in 0.01 M EDTA (ethylenediamine tetraacetic acid, pH 5.0, RSC 0.78) and centrifuged at 41,300 × g for 20 min for sedimentation of insoluble aggregates. The supernatant was dialyzed against 1 liter of 72 mM EDTA (pH 5.0, RSC 0.08) for 3.5 hr in the cold. The precipitate was washed once in the same concentration of EDTA and once in 0.07 M NaCl before being redissolved in 7 ml of 0.75 M NaCl. This final solution of purified Clq was centrifuged at 41,300 × g for 20 min for sedimentation of insoluble aggregates; the clear supernatant was either used immediately for electron microscopy or stored at 4°C in 0.75 M NaCl, or fixed in a final concentration of 0.1% formaldehyde.

Purity of Preparation. The purity of the preparations was checked by radial immunodiffusion in individual agarose plates, each containing an antiserum to Clq, IgG, IgM, or IgA (3). By this method the preparation was shown to contain about 95% Clq, contaminated with 5% IgG, IgM, and IgA. Precipitation with soluble, heat-denatured IgG (heated at 63°C for 12 min) at an RSC of 0.112 indicated that 85–90% of the Clq was capable of binding to IgG. Heating aliquots at

56°C for 30 min completely destroyed the IgG binding capacity.

Electron Microscopy; Dilution of Clq with Glutamine Synthetase. The concentration of protein that was optimum for visualizing individual Clq molecules by negative staining was very low and resulted in unsatisfactory preparations. To overcome this difficulty, the routine was established of diluting Clq into a solution containing the enzyme, glutamine synthetase (EC 6.3.1.2; derived from *Escherichia coli*, a kind gift from Dr. Richard Miller). This relatively large molecule provided the increment of protein needed routinely to obtain excellent negative stains. The glutamine synthetase molecules were stored at 4°C in 30% ammonium sulfate at a concentration of 7.4 mg/ml. Immediately before use as a diluent for Clq, the enzyme was diluted 1–1000 in distilled water. When the unfixed enzyme by itself was stained in 1% uranyl acetate, no subunits were seen and only rarely were partially disintegrated molecules observed. Mixing the two molecules together not only resulted in excellent negative stains but also provided each photomicrograph with a built-in magnification calibration. Valentine *et al.* (6), who thoroughly characterized the ultrastructure of glutamine synthetase, found the molecule to be 14 nm (140 Å) in diameter when stained with sodium silicotungstate. Our measurements show the molecule consistently to be 16 nm (160 Å) in diameter, the higher value probably resulting from the shallower pool of negative stain produced by uranyl acetate.

To prepare Clq molecules for examination in the electron microscope, samples were diluted with 0.75 M NaCl to a concentration of 2–10 μg/ml in polyethylene tubes. Aliquots were mixed 1:1 with diluted glutamine synthetase and droplets were placed on carbon-coated collodion membranes supported on 400-mesh copper grids and allowed to remain for 3 min. The droplets were removed with filter paper and immediately replaced with several droplets of 1% aqueous uranyl acetate (pH 4.2) in a rinse–stain step. The uranyl acetate was allowed to dry, and the preparations were examined and photographed in a Siemens Elmiskop 101 electron microscope at initial magnifications of 60,000 and 80,000 by use of a 50-μm objective aperture and 80 kV accelerating voltage. The magnification of the instrument was checked by making a series of photographs of the 2.5-nm (25-Å) spacing in crystals of Indanthrene Olive TWP (a generous gift from Dr. L. W. Labaw) concurrent with the photographs of the molecules of Clq (7).

RESULTS

The Clq molecule was present only in those preparations

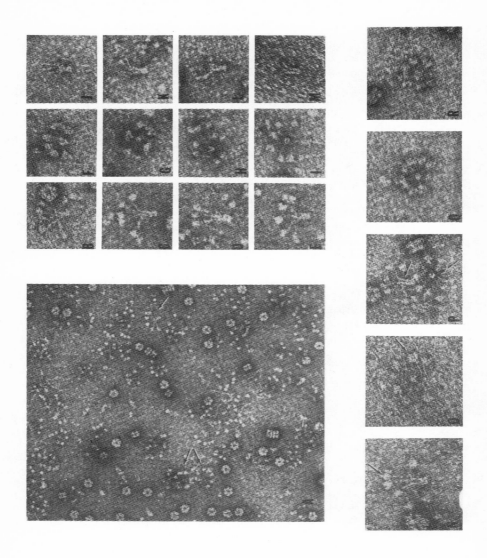

FIG. 1. (*A*) Survey view of negatively stained Clq molecules and "marker" molecules of glutamine synthetase, 16 nm (160 Å) in diameter. The 6-nm (60-Å) terminal subunits of Clq are easily recognized, but very few whole Clq molecules are present because 1 week elapsed between isolation and preparation for electron microscopy. A pair of *arrows* points to top views of whole molecules, a single *arrow* points to the side view of whole molecule. ×200,000. (*B–E*) Side views of Clq molecules showing attachment of terminal subunits to central subunit by connecting strands; *D* shows a partial molecule. ×400,000. (*F–I*) Top views of Clq showing disposition of terminal subunits around the central subunit. Note the varying morphology of this view of the central subunit. ×400,000. (*J–M*) Central subunits with attached connecting strands. ×400,000. (*N*) Side view of Clq showing division of terminal subunit into two unequal parts. Observe attachment of connecting strand to larger of the two subdivisions (*arrow*). Note also that the central subunit appears to be divided into two parts longitudinally. ×500,000. (*O*) Top view of Clq showing another divided terminal subunit with the connecting strand attached to the larger component (*arrow*) ×500,000. (*P*) Side and top views of the two Clq molecules illustrating the cleft in the central subunit (*arrows*). Note the similarity between the central subunit in side view (*solid arrow*) and the isolated subunit in Fig. 1 *M*. ×400,000. (*Q, R*) Top views of molecule showing some connecting strands and illustrating difficulty in counting number of terminal subunits in this aspect. ×400,000.

demonstrated to have biological activity. The heat-denatured Clq appeared in electron micrographs as agglutinated masses with no distinctive shape or size. In preparations containing biologically active Clq, on the other hand, individual molecules and parts of molecules could be readily distinguished-The survey view (Fig. 1A) of Clq molecules dispersed among the distinctive glutamine synthetase molecules is a study in contrast. Glutamine synthetase is a sturdy molecule, its twelve subunits always appear as a stack of two hexagons; Clq is clearly not only extremely labile, in that pieces of the molecule outnumber whole molecules, but it is also extremely flexible since the whole molecule rarely presents exactly the same aspect. *Arrows* (Fig. 1A) point to two complete molecules viewed from the "top" and to one complete molecule viewed from the "side".

Viewed from the side at higher magnification (Fig. 1B–E), the molecule is seen to consist of six terminal subunits linked by tenuous connections to a stalk-like central subunit. Partial molecules Fig. 1D, consisting of the central subunit and 2–5 terminal subunits with connecting strands, are not uncommon. Viewed from the top, (Fig. 1F–I, Q, and R) the terminal subunits are usually less clearly delineated and frequently appear to be more than 6 in number; the connecting subunits are normally not seen, although they are clearly present in some aspects (Fig. 1O, R). The terminal subunits are most frequently disposed in a semicircle about the central subunit; very rarely they form an equally-spaced circle.

Central subunits, devoid of terminal subunits but sometimes bearing connecting strands, are fairly numerous (Fig. 1J–M). Viewed from the top, (Fig. 1F–I) the central subunit appears to be solid, "V"- or ring-shaped, suggesting that this subunit is subdivided, a possibility that is strengthened by some aspects of this subunit in side-view. Compare the morphology of the isolated central subunit in Fig. 1M with that of the whole molecule in Fig. 1P (*arrow*); they appear to be identical in having a cleft that runs almost the full length of the subunit. Furthermore, in the top view of the molecule, Fig. 1P (*broken arrow*), the central subunit has a "C"-shape that would indicate correspondence to such a cleft. There is evidence that the terminal subunits are also divided into two smaller components, which appear to be unequal in size, and that the connecting strands appear to be attached to the larger of the two (Fig. 1N and O, *arrows*). The further division of the terminal subunits would explain the fact that frequently there seem to be more than six of them.

The diameter of the molecule measured across the span of the terminal subunits in either top or side-view, lies between 27 and 38.5 nm (270 and 385 Å), indicating that although the molecule is flexible, there are limits beyond which it

142

cannot be distorted. The height of the molecule in side view measures between 28 and 33 nm (280 and 330 Å). The terminal subunits measure between 5 and 7.5 nm (50 and 75 Å) and appear to be somewhat longer than they are broad. In the two cases illustrated in Fig. 1N and O, where division of the terminal subunit into unequal parts is clearly visible, the larger and smaller units measure, respectively, 5 × 6.5 nm (50 × 65 Å) and 2.5 × 7 nm (25 × 70 Å). The connecting strands measure about 1.5 nm (15 Å) in width and between 10–13 nm (100–130 Å) in length. The central subunit measures between 3 and 6 nm (30 and 60 Å) across and about 10–12.5 nm (100–125 Å) in length.

DISCUSSION

The fragility of the Clq molecule has made its ultrastructural characterization extraordinarily difficult. In order to obtain a large number of intact molecules, we found it essential to make preparations of Clq for electron microscopy immediately after its isolation from freshly drawn blood. The freshly isolated molecules do not resemble in size or shape those described by Svehag and Bloth (5); whereas they found that fixation in formaldehyde stabilized the molecule, we found no difference in morphology between fixed and unfixed molecules. The Clq molecule, as we view it, consists of three distinct parts that we called terminal subunits, connecting strands, and a central subunit. Each terminal subunit is further divided into a large and a small subunit; morphologic evidence suggests that the central subunit also is divided longitudinally into two parts. In the intact molecule, six connecting strands join the terminal subunits by their larger subdivision to the central subunit. This morphologic concept of the molecule is compatible with recent chemical data (Yonemasu and Stroud, submitted for publication) that demonstrate that Clq may be dissociated into three electrophoretically distinct, covalently bonded subunits, multiples of which make up the whole molecule, or into two, noncovalently linked subunits of unequal molecular weight (estimated to be 60,000 and 42,000) that appear in a molar ratio of 3:1. It is conceivable that each terminal subunit and its connecting strand corresponds to the heavier, noncovalent moiety, and each part of the central subunit corresponds to the lighter one, but at present we cannot definitely correlate the morphologic subunits with their chemical counterparts.

Perhaps the most unusual feature of Clq is the delicacy of its structure. The strands connecting the terminal subunits to the central subunit possibly consist of single polypeptide chains, since they clearly are finer than the paired heavy chains of the IgM molecule. The structure of Clq also reflects its low molecular weight of about 400,000, as compared

143

with a molecular weight about 900,000 for the denser, more compact IgM (8, 9); in some other respects, however, the two molecules are surprisingly similar. Both have radial subunits attached at a central locus, and their overall dimensions are approximately the same, i.e., about 35 nm (350 Å). Thus, the shape of the Clq molecule, like that of IgM, may reflect its function: both molecules have the possibility for flexibility built into their structure and both molecules act as physical links in the interacting molecular systems of which they are a part.

This research was supported in part by grants from NIH and the Veterans Administration.

1. Müller-Eberhard, H. J. & Kunkel, H. G. (1961) "Isolation of a Thermolabile Serum Protein Which Precipitates γ-Globulin Aggregates and Participates in Immune Hemolysis", *Proc. Soc. Exp. Biol. Med.* **106**, 291–297.
2. Müller-Eberhard, H. J., (1968) "Chemistry and Reaction Mechanisms of Complement", *Advan. Immunol.* **8**, 1–80.
3. Yonemasu, K. & Stroud, R. M. (1971) "Clq: Rapid Purification Method for Preparation of Monospecific Antisera and for Biochemical Studies", *J. Immunol.* **106**, 304–413.
4. Yonemasu, K., Stroud, R. M., Niedermeier, W. & Butler, W. T. (1971) "Chemical Studies on Clq; a Modulator of Immunoglobulin Biology", *Biochem. Biophys. Res. Commun.* **43**, 1388–1394.
5. Svehag, S-E. & Bloth, B. (1970) "The Ultrastructure of Human Clq", *Acta Pathol. Microbiol. Scand.* [B] **78**, 260–262.
6. Valentine, R. C., Shapiro, B. M. & Stadtman, E. R. (1968) "Regulation of Glutamine Synthetase. XII Electron Microscopy of the Enzyme from *Escherichia coli*", *Biochemistry* **7**, 2143–2152.
7. Labaw, L. W. (1964) "Preparation of a 25-A Spacing Crystal for Magnification Calibration above 18,000 X", *J. Appl. Phys.* **35**, 3076.
8. Chesebro, B., Bloth, B. & Svehag, S-E. (1968) "The Ultrastructure of Normal and Pathological IgM Immunoglobulins", *J. Exp. Med.* **127**, 399–410.
9. Shelton, E. & McIntire, K. R. (1970) "Ultrastructure of the γM Immunoglobulin Molecule", *J. Mol. Biol.* **47**, 595–597.

Genetic Aspects

Hereditary C2 Deficiency with Some Manifestations of Systemic Lupus Erythematosus

V. AGNELLO, M. M. E. DE BRACCO AND H. G. KUNKEL

Thus far hereditary deficiency of the second component of complement (C2) has been described in four kindreds (1–4). The homozygous individuals showed marked depression of total serum hemolytic complement, but were found to have relatively normal immune adherence and bactericidal function of their sera and were all clinically healthy individuals (1–5). These findings have raised considerable question about the role of the intact complement system in biologic defense mechanisms of man. The present paper reports studies on a fifth kindred which manifests the C2 deficiency trait and the first in which the deficiency is associated with a disease state. The proposita, homozygous for the trait, has a lupus-like syndrome and a clinical course which has been marked by severe recurrent skin rash.

MATERIALS AND METHODS

Serum samples were obtained from clotted blood, flash frozen and stored at $-50°C$. Samples were thawed once. The total hemolytic complement titer (CH_{50}) was determined by the method of Kent and Fife (6). Stoichiometric titrations of complement component hemolytic activity (SFU) were performed as previously described (4, 7–9). Serum protein concentrations of complement components and C1 inhibitor were determined by radial immunodiffusion. Monospecific antiserum to C2 was provided by Doctors M. Polley and

[1] This investigation was supported by United States Public Health Service Grant AM 04761 and Grant RR-102 from the General Clinical Research Centers Program of the Division of Research Resources, National Institutes of Health.

H. Müller-Eberhard. Immune adherence assays were done by the method of Gewurz *et al.* (5). Serum opsonic activity studies against *Escherichia coli* and *Staphylococcus aureus* were performed by Dr. R. Williams (10). Immunofluorescence studies, using methods previously described (11), were performed by Dr. D. Koffler.

Medical history of the proposita. The proposita, a 55-year-old Caucasian female, developed an erythematous scaly rash on the face, neck and forearms in September 1967 following extensive sun exposure. The rash cleared slowly with the administration of topical corticosteroid cream treatment. In January 1971, the facial rash recurred without unusual exposure to the sun. Two months later she was hospitalized because of progression of the rash, generalized arthralgias and low grade fever. Past medical history included:. varicella, variola and mumps virus infections in childhood without complications, multiple episodes of otitis media in childhood resulting in perforated tympanic membranes, pneumonitis of the left lung in 1965 and recurrent episodes of acute bronchitis.

On the admission the only physical abnormalities were perforated tympanic membranes and an extensive erythematous, raised rash over face, arms, legs and back. Laboratory findings included: hemoglobin 10.7%, white blood cells (WBC) 4300/mm³, erythrocyte sedimentation rate 90 mm/hr, blood urea nitrogen 9 mg%, total serum protein 6.4 g%, γ globulin 1.44 g% and ASO titer 1:400. An initial 24-hour urine protein was 0.8 g; subsequent determinations were within normal limits. Creatinine clearance was 105 ml/min. The remainder of the urinalysis was unremarkable. The electrocardiogram was normal. Chest x-ray showed old pleural thickening at the left lung base. The rash cleared completely in 4 weeks with topical corticosteroid therapy. The arthralgias and fever subsided during hospitalization without systemic therapy.

RESULTS

Serum levels of C2 and total hemolytic complement on 13 members of Family S are shown in Table I. Individuals with C2 deficiency were

TABLE I

*Serum hemolytic complement and C2 titers of
individual members of the kindred*

Individual	Age	CH_{50}	C2 SFU/ml
	years	*u/ml*	
I, 2	80	175	570
II, 1	56	250	1575
II, 2	55	<10	<1
III, 1	28	243	1260
III, 2	29	154	662
III, 3	27	156	645
III, 4	30	227	1386
IV, 1	3	204	1197
IV, 2	1	225	1197
IV, 3	5	181	1197
IV, 4	3	170	662
IV, 5	1	162	630
Normal range		150–250	1000–1600

found in each of four generations (Fig. 1) and
the segregation of this trait is consistent with the
Mendelian mode of inheritance which has been
reported by Klemperer, Austen, Rosen and others
(1–4). Serum of the proposita (II, 2) had no demonstrable total complement hemolytic activity
and no detectable C2 by either hemolytic assay
or immunoligic analysis. Addition of 2000 SFU
of isolated guinea pig C2 to the deficient serum
restored the hemolytic activity to normal
(CH_{50} 164). There was no evidence of a circulating
serum C2 inhibitory factor in the proposita since
the titer of C2 hemolytic activity in normal
serum was unaffected by addition of the C2-
deficient serum. The heterozygous individuals
were recognized by the presence in their serum of
approximately 50% of the normal C2 values;
however, total hemolytic complement activity
was not proportionately depressed but was at
the lower range of the normal limits as has been
reported previously in these cases (4).

Studies on other early serum complement components in the proposita (Table II) showed the
C2 deficiency to be selective. Late component
complement activity, C3 through C9, was tested
with EAC142 intermediate cells and was found

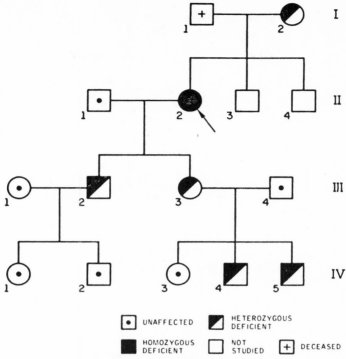

I

II

III

IV

- ⊡ UNAFFECTED
- ◩ HETEROZYGOUS DEFICIENT
- ■ HOMOZYGOUS DEFICIENT
- ☐ NOT STUDIED
- ⊞ DECEASED

Figure 1. Pedigree of Family S.

to be normal. The C1 esterase inhibitor was significantly above normal levels. The complement-mediated biologic functions of the serum which were tested, immune adherence and opsonic activity, were normal.

Clinically, the recurrent rash which the proposita has had over the past 4 years appeared typical of systemic lupus erythematosus (SLE). Serologic studies gave evidence for SLE. The LE cell test was positive; the antinuclear fluorescence test was $2+$; strong precipitins to nucleoprotein were present; antibodies in low titer to DNA (1:16) and heat-denatured DNA (1:16) were also present transiently. In addition, low titers of rheumatoid factor were present. Antibodies to synthetic double stranded RNA (poly A·U) and soluble nuclear extract antigens were not present in this case.

In contrast to the serologic findings, studies of a biopsy of the skin rash did not show the typical

TABLE II
*Serum complement component studies
in the proposita*

	Proposita	Normal Range
C1 SFU/ml[a]	103,000	100,000–250,000
C1q μg/ml	220	130–210
C1r % normal	100	82–115
C1s μg/ml	27.6	23–35
C4 SFU/ml[a]	182,000	90,000–200,000
C4 μg/ml	460	390–654
C2 SFU/ml[a]	<1	1,000–1,600
C2 μg/ml	<0.5	8–12
C3 mg %	187.5	104–148
C1 inhibitor % normal	170	85–110

[a] Hemolytic titrations; all other determinations by radial immunodiffusion.

pathology of SLE. Immunofluorescent staining showed no deposits of immunoglobulins, or the C1q and C3 components of complement. Light microscopy, however, showed changes consistent with those found in SLE; edema and infiltration of lymphocytes and neutrophils were present focally in the upper dermis associated with basal layer degeneration of adjacent epidermis. No vasculitis was present. Immunofluorescence studies of a renal biopsy failed to show deposits of immunoglobulin, C1q or C3.

The heterozygous C2-deficient members of the kindred showed no clinical or serologic abnormalities.

DISCUSSION

The affected individual studied in this paper had a clinical picture consistent with SLE with a positive LE cell test and other serologic characteristics of this disease. The skin rash, which was the dominant clinical manifestation, appeared typical of SLE although biopsy studies failed to demonstrate immunoglobulin deposits at the dermal-epidermal junction as are usually found (12). Fluorescent antibody studies failed to show any γ globulin deposits in a kidney biopsy which is extremely unusual for SLE patients (11). It is possible that these atypical features relate in part to the extremely low complement levels. Alternatively, the lack of immunoglobulin and complement deposits in the skin and kidney may reflect an absence of circulating immune complexes. In support of this possibility was the finding that there was no depression of C1 or C4 as is found in the presence of circulating complexes (13).

The highest prevalence for SLE in a recent study was 134.4/million (14). While the exact prevalence of the homozygous state for C2 deficiency is not known, experience in our laboratory primarily with hospital patients indicates only the one case in 10,000 studied. Another estimate can be made from the studies of Hässig and colleagues (15). Among 41,082 Swiss army recruits they found 14 individuals with deficiency in serum hemolytic complement. Assuming all of these were due to C2 deficiency, which is unlikely, the probability that both SLE and the homozygous C2 deficiency state would be found in the same individual is of the order of 1 in 20 million. It appears unlikely then that the association of C2 deficiency and the manifestations of SLE were coincidental. Also, it appears likely that two other similar cases have been encountered. Pickering and associates (16), in a description of unusual complement alteration in glomerulonephritis, mention a patient with selective C2 deficiency (apparently not hereditary) who showed skin rash and other manifestations of SLE. Sussman, Jones and Lachmann[2] have also studied a patient with selective C2 deficiency who has recurrent skin rash; however, the kindred of this case has not been studied as yet.

While the association of two rare conditions does not necessarily indicate a causal relation, such a possibility must be strongly suspected. This patient showed evidence of increased infections for a number of years. The possibility that SLE has an infectious basis, particularly viral, currently is a widely held concept (17, 18). A not unreasonable hypothesis would be that in the setting of virtually absent complement the likelihood of proliferation of such an agent may be increased and result in the clinical picture of

[2] Personal communication from Doctors Sussman, Jones and Lachmann.

SLE in some but not necessarily all such C2-deficient individuals.

Acknowledgment. We would like to thank Doctors M. Polley and H. Müller-Eberhard for their gifts of C2 antisera, Dr. R. Williams for performing the opsonic studies, and Dr. C. L. Christian for helpful discussions. We also thank Miss Liling Shen for her excellent technical assistance.

SUMMARY

A family with hereditary C2 deficiency was studied. The proposita, homozygous for this trait, showed certain clinical and serologic manifestations of systemic lupus erythematosus which included a widespread skin rash and a positive LE cell test.

REFERENCES

1. Klemperer, M. R., Woodworth, H. C., Rosen, F. S. and Austen, K. F., J. Clin. Invest., *45:* 880, 1966.
2. Klemperer, M. R., Austen, K. F. and Rosen, F. S., J. Immunol., *98:* 72, 1967.
3. Cooper, N. R., Ten Bensel, R. and Kohler, P. F., J. Immunol., *101:* 1176, 1968.
4. Ruddy, S., Klemperer, M. R., Rosen, F. S., Austen, K. F. and Kumate, J., Immunology, *18:* 943, 1970.
5. Gewurz, H., Pickering, R. J., Muschel, L. H., Mergenhagen, S. E. and Good, R. A., Lancet, *2:* 356, 1966.
6. Kent, J. F. and Fife, E. H., Am. J. Trop. Med. Hyg., *12:* 103, 1963.
7. Borsos, T. and Rapp, H. J., J. Immunol., *91:* 851, 1963.
8. Borsos, T., Rapp, H. J. and Mayer, M. M., J. Immunol., *87:* 310, 1961.
9. Ruddy, S. and Austen, K. F., J. Immunol., *99:* 1162, 1967.
10. Williams, R. C., Jr., and Quie, P. G., J. Immunol., *106:* 51, 1971.
11. Koffler, D., Agnello, V., Carr, R. I. and Kunkel, H. G., Am. J. Pathol., *56:* 305, 1969.
12. Tan, E. M. and Kunkel, H. G., Arthritis Rheum., *9:* 37, 1966.
13. Kohler, P. F. and Ten Bensel, R., Clin. Exp. Immunol., *4:* 191, 1969.
14. Siegel, M., Holley, H. L. and Lee, S. L., Arthritis Rheum., *13:* 802, 1970.

15. Hässig, V. A., Borel, J. F., Ammann, P.,
Thöni, M. and Bütler, R., Pathol. Microbiol., *27:* 542, 1964.
16. Pickering, R. J., Michael, A. F., Jr., Herd-
man, R. C., Good, R. A. and Gewurz, H., J.
Pediatr. *78:* 30, 1971.
17. Gyorkey, F., Min, K. W., Sincovics, J. G. and
Gyorkey, P., N. Engl. J. Med., *280:* 333,
1969.
18. Christian, C. L., N. Engl. J. Med., *280:* 878,
1969.

HEMOLYTIC EFFICIENCIES OF GENETIC VARIANTS
OF HUMAN C3[1]

HARVEY R. COLTEN AND CHESTER A. ALPER

The hemolytic efficiency of the genetic variants of the third component of complement (C3), native C3 in serum and highly purified C3 were estimated. The specific hemolytic activities of each of the partially purified variants were similar to that of C3 in whole serum but only about 20% that of highly purified C3. In the highly purified preparation, approximately 300 C3 molecules were bound for each hemolytic site.

The third component of complement (C3) exhibits extensive genetic structural polymorphism (1, 2). At least 14 variants, detected by electrophoresis of whole serum, have been identified (3). These genetic markers have been used to demonstrate the failure of C3 to cross the placenta (2, 4) and to provide evidence that the liver is the primary, if not sole, site of C3 synthesis *in vivo* (5). Although the complement activities of several of the variants have been crudely assessed (6), no truly quantitative assays have yet been reported.

In the present study, the specific activities of C3 $F_{1.1}$, F_1, $F_{0.85}$, $F_{0.8}$, F, S, $S_{0.6}$ and S_1 have been determined. All the C3 variants were found to have similar hemolytic activities. The specific hemolytic activities of the partially purified variants were similar to that of C3 in whole serum but lower than the specific activity of highly purified C3.

[1] This work was supported by Grants AI-05877 and AM-13855 from the United States Public Health Service.

Sera. Blood samples from individuals either homozygous for the common alleles, $C3^F$ or $C3^S$, or heterozygous for $C3^F$ or $C3^S$ and a rare C3 allele were allowed to clot for about 1 hr at room temperature. Serum was then obtained by centrifugation and stored at $-80°C$. Samples were thawed immediately before analysis.

Preparative prolonged agarose gel electrophoresis. Prolonged agarose gel electrophoresis was carried out as described previously (1). The same sample was introduced into each of 5 sample slots. After the electrophoretic separation was completed, the C3 area of the gel was sliced into 1.2-mm segments (7). Each slice was eluted separately into 0.1 ml dextrose Veronal-buffered saline ($\mu = 0.075$, pH 7.35) containing 1.5×10^{-4} M Ca^{2+} and 10^{-3} M Mg^{2+} (VBS-D) (8) at 4°C overnight. To assess the loss of C3 activity during the elution procedure, samples were allowed to diffuse into gels prepared for, but not subjected to, electrophoresis for the usual duration of electrophoretic separation (6 hr). The gel around the origin was sliced and eluted as described above.

C3 determinations. The concentration of hemolytically effective C3 molecules in each sample was determined by modification of the method given in reference nine by using functionally purified human complement components. Partially purified human C2, C5, C6, C7, C8 and C9 were purchased from Cordis Laboratories (Miami, Fla.). Buffers and red cell intermediates were prepared as given in reference eight. C3 was purified by the method given in reference 10; human C1 by zonal centrifugation (11).

Hemolytic efficiency of C3 was estimated in the following manner: purified C3 was labeled with ^{125}I by the iodine monochloride method (12). One-milliliter aliquots of dilutions of the ^{125}I-labeled C3 were each incubated at 30°C for 30 min with 1 ml of $EAC\overline{14}$ (1×10^9 cells/ml) and and 1 ml of VBS-D containing human C2 (1000 effective molecules/ml). The cell suspensions were then washed in VBS-D four times and the radioactivity of the cell buttons and the washes was counted in a Packard Gamma Scintillation Spectrometer (Packard Instrument Co., Inc., Down-

155

er's Grove, Ill.). Controls were handled in the same way except that C2 was omitted. Before the cell mixtures were washed, a 60-μl aliquot of each was removed and diluted 1:13 in VBS-D. The number of hemolytically active C3 molecules

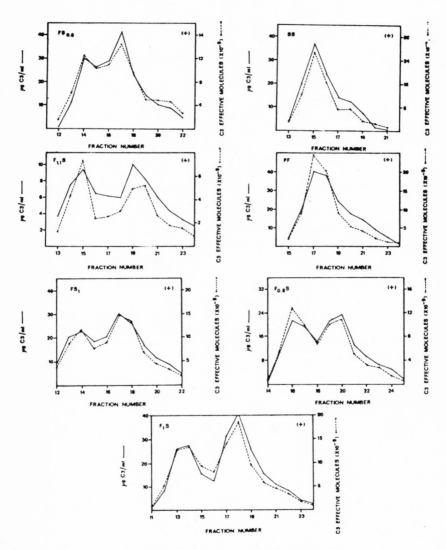

Figure 1. Hemolytic and immunochemical assay of genetically determined C3 variants separated by preparative electrophoresis in agarose gel.

per cell was then estimated by adding partially purified C2 and C5-C9 and measuring the extent of lysis in the usual manner (9). Specific C3 activity in whole serum and isolated variants was calculated as effective C3 molecules per μg of C3 protein. C3 concentration was also determined in all the samples by an electroimmunochemical technique (13) with monospecific antiserum to C3 prepared in rabbits.

RESULTS

Specific activities of C3 variants. C3 hemolytic activity closely paralleled C3 protein concentration in electrophoretic fractions of all variant-containing sera, as shown in Figure 1. Most patterns contained, in addition to the two major C3 bands, an anodal shoulder of both C3 protein and functionally active C3 molecules.

Specific activities for each of the C3 variants studied are given in Table I. Specific activities were calculated from the average C3 protein content and hemolytic activity in two to four fractions from each of the electrophoretically separated peaks. It is evident that the activities of the rare variants, C3 $F_{1.1}$, F_1, $F_{0.85}$, $S_{0.6}$ and S_1, are similar to those of the common variants in each serum. The specific activity of whole serum C3 was on the average 6.9×10^8 effective molecules/μg, whereas that of the same sample subjected to "mock electrophoresis" and elution was on the average 4.5×10^8 effective molecules/μg C3.

TABLE I

Specific C3 hemolytic activity in several genetic variants

Serum C3 Type	Hemolytically Effective C3 Molecules ($\times 10^{-8}$)/μg						
	S_1	$S_{0.6}$	S	F	$F_{0.8}$	F_1	$F_{1.1}$
$F_{1.1}S$			5.8				5.4
F_1S			4.9			4.5	
$F_{0.8}S$			5.7		4.5		
FF				5.3			
SS			5.9				
$FS_{0.6}$		4.0		3.7			
FS_1	4.6			4.8			

Hemolytic efficiency of highly purified C3. The results of this experiment, summarized in Table II, show that approximately 23% of the ^{125}I-labeled C3 was taken up on $EAC\overline{142}$. In contrast, only 0.1% was taken up on $EAC\overline{14}$. The preparation contained 374 μg of C3/ml or 1.22 $\times$ 10^{15} molecules/ml (assuming a m.w. of 185,000 for C3), 22.5% of which (2.75 $\times$ 10^{14} molecules/ml) were bound to the cells. There were 9.6 $\times$ 10^{11} effective molecules of C3/ml as measured by the hemolytic assay. Therefore, under the conditions of this hemolytic assay, 290 to 300 molecules of ^{125}I-labeled C3/cell were bound for each hemolytic site.

DISCUSSION

The results indicate that of the C3 variants studied, both common and rare, all had approximately the same specific C3 hemolytic activities. This suggests that the structural features responsible for human C3 polymorphism do not affect the functionally active sites of the molecule. Since the polymorphism probably reflects minor substitutions in a large molecule with an approximate m.w. of 185,000 (14), the failure of such substitutions to interfere with function is not surprising. Similarly, genetic variants of transferrin had comparable abilities to bind and release iron (15). Most of the many known hemoglobin variants are likewise normal in function (16).

The anodally-migrating gene-specific minor C3 components (1, 2) have here been shown to possess approximately the same specific functional activity as the major C3 proteins. Therefore, whatever the molecular basis for these minor gene-specific components, it does not affect the hemolytic function of C3.

It is interesting that C3 S_1, which appears to bind more Ca^{2+} than the other variants of this study (17), has the same specific activity as the latter. The relationship of Ca^{2+}-binding to the function of C3 remains obscure.

Cooper, Polley and Müller-Eberhard have estimated that approximately 100 to 200 bound C3 molecules are required to generate a hemolytic site (18). Our data confirm their findings. Interestingly, if one assumes that the proportion of C3 in whole serum bound to $EAC\overline{142}$ is similar

TABLE II

Hemolytic efficiency of C3

Dilution of C3	Radioactivity (CPM)[a]			Immunochemical Analysis			Hemolytic Effective mol. C3 ($\times 10^{-9}$)/ml	C3 Mol./Hemolytic Site
	Total	Uptake on EAC142[b]	% uptake	Total C3 (μg/ml)	Total C3 molecules ($\times 10^{-11}$)/ml	Uptake on EAC142 C3 mol. ($\times 10^{-11}$)/ml		
1:400	36,890	8,300	22.5	0.93[c]	30.2	6.8	2.29	296
1:800	18,000	4,370	23.5	0.465[c]	15.1	3.5	1.20	290

[a] CPM = counts per minute.
[b] At 1:400 dilution of C3 preparation, uptake on $\overline{EAC14}$ = 38 CPM or 0.1% of total radioactivity.
[c] Calculated from C3 protein in undiluted sample (374 μg/ml).

159

to that of purified preparations, the calculated hemolytic efficiency of C3 in whole serum was only 20% of that of isolated C3. This difference may be due to either specific (C3 inactivator) or nonspecific inhibitory factors present in serum that interfere with the detection of hemolytically active C3.

Acknowledgments. Miss Lillian Watson and Miss Nabuko Sugimoto provided expert technical assistance. Dr. Fred S. Rosen collaborated in the preparation of the purified C3.

REFERENCES

1. Alper, C. A. and Propp, R. P., J. Clin. Invest., *47:* 2181, 1968.
2. Azen, E. A. and Smithies, O., Science, *162:* 905, 1968.
3. Alper, C. A., Progr. Immunol. *1:* 609, 1971.
4. Propp, R. P. and Alper, C. A., Science, *162:* 672, 1968.
5. Alper, C. A., Johnson, A. M., Birtch, A. G. and Moore, F. D., Science, *163:* 286, 1969.
6. Alper, C. A. and Rosen, F. S., in *Advances in Immunology,* Edited by F. J. Dixon and H. G. Kunkel, Vol. 14, p. 251, Academic Press, New York, 1971.
7. Alper, C. A., Abramson, N., Johnston, R. B., Jr., Jandl, J. H. and Rosen, F. S., J. Clin. Invest., *49:* 1975, 1970.
8. Rapp, H. J. and Borsos, T., *Molecular Basis of Complement Action,* p. 75, Appleton-Century-Crofts, New York, 1970.
9. Nelson, R. A., Jr., Jensen, J., Gigli, I. and Tamura, N., Immunochemistry, *3:* 111, 1966.
10. Nilsson, U. R. and Müller-Eberhard, H. J., J. Exp. Med., *122:* 277, 1965.
11. Colten, H. R., Bond, H. E., Borsos, T. and Rapp, H. J., J. Immunol., *103:* 862, 1969.
12. McFarlane, A. S., Nature, *182:* 53, 1958.
13. Laurell, C.-B., Anal. Biochem., *15:* 45, 1966.
14. Müller-Eberhard, H. J., Ann. Rev. Biochem., *38:* 389, 1969.
15. Turnbull, A. and Giblett, E. R., J. Lab. Clin. Med., *57:* 450, 1961.
16. Giblett, E. R., *Genetic Markers in Human Blood,* p. 370, Blackwell, Oxford, 1969.

17. Alper, C. A., in *Protides of the Biological Fluids*, Vol. 17, p. 295, Edited by H. Peeters, Pergamon Press, Oxford, 1970.

18. Cooper, N. R., Polley, M. J. and Müller-Eberhard, H. J., in *Immunological Diseases*, 2nd Ed., Vol. 1, p. 289, Edited by M. Samter and D. W. Talmage, Little, Brown, 1971.

Biosynthesis of the Second (C2) and Fourth (C4) Components of Complement *in vitro* by Tissues Isolated from Guinea-Pigs with Genetically Determined C4 Deficiency*

H. R. Colten and M. M. Frank

Summary. Tissues and cells isolated from guinea-pigs homozygous for a genetically determined deficiency of the fourth (C4) component of complement failed to synthesize C4 and synthesized C2 at a rate approximately 40 per cent of normal. These abnormalities in the biosynthesis of C2 and C4 persisted up to four weeks in tissue culture. Tissues and cells from heterozygous C4-deficient animals produced C4 at a rate intermediate between normal and that of the homozygous deficient. These observations demonstrate that the reduced serum concentrations of C2 and C4 in C4-deficient guinea-pigs can be accounted for by abnormalities in biosynthesis and are probably not the result of hypercatabolism of these proteins.

INTRODUCTION

Methods now available for studies of the biosynthesis of serum complement (C) components *in vitro* have made it possible to identify the sites of synthesis of most of the individual complement components (Colten and Wyatt, 1971). Interest in this area has been stimulated largely by the discovery of genetic abnormalities of the complement system in man (Donaldson and Evans, 1963; Klemperer, Woodworth, Rosen and Austen 1966; Alper, Propp, Klemperer and Rosen, 1969) and experimental animals (Rosenberg and Tachibana, 1962; Rother, Rother, Müller-Eberhard and Nilsson, 1966; Ellman, Green and Frank, 1970). The methods developed in the course of the studies of complement biosynthesis *in vitro* provide a direct approach to the problem of localizing the biochemical lesions responsible for genetic abnormalities of complement production. An opportunity to study a genetic abnormality of complement biosynthesis was made possible by the availability of several animals from a strain of guinea-pigs with a genetically determined deficiency of C4 (Ellman, Green and Frank, 1970). Breeding experiments, as well as measurements of C4 in the sera of homozygous and heterozygous deficient animals, have established that this abnormality is inherited as an autosomal recessive trait. An interesting feature of this strain is that, in addition to the total deficiency of C4, the content of the second (C2) component of C is approximately one-half normal in the sera of most homozygous C4-deficient animals

* Supported in part by USPHS Grant No. AI–05877–08.

162

(Frank, May, Gaither and Ellman, 1971). At the time this observation was reported, it was not known whether the decreased levels of C2 were a consequence of increased catabolism or decreased synthesis of the C2 protein.

In the experiments reported here, liver, spleen and peritoneal exudates from homozygous deficient, heterozygous deficient, and normal guinea-pigs were cultured *in vitro* and the capacity of each to synthesize C2 and C4 was determined. Cells isolated from homozygous deficient animals did not produce C4 *in vitro*, and cells from heterozygous deficient animals produced less than normal amounts of C4. C2 synthesis by cells and tissues isolated from homozygous C4 deficient animals was less than normal, accounting for the reduced serum levels of C2 in these animals. In each case, the relative reduction in rates of *in vitro* C2 and C4 synthesis by homozygous and heterozygous deficient cells correlated well with the reduced serum levels of the corresponding component. These abnormalities of complement biosynthesis persisted up to four weeks after isolating the cells *in vitro*.

MATERIALS AND METHODS

The preparation of sheep erythrocytes (E) rabbit antibody to boiled stromata of E (A) and the cell intermediates EAC1 and EAC14 have been described by Rapp and Borsos, (1970). Details of preparation of veronal-buffered saline (VBS), veronal-buffered saline-sucrose (VBS-sucrose, $\mu = 0.065$), and ethylenediaminetetraacetate (EDTA) buffer (0.01 M, pH 7.5), as well as methods for the isolation of partially purified guinea-pig C1 and C2, are also given by Rapp and Borsos (1970). Haemolytic titrations of C2 and C4 were performed as given in (Opferkuch, Rapp, Colten and Borsos, 1971) using rat CEDTA (rat serum diluted 1/5 in EDTA buffer).

Homozygous and heterozygous C4-deficient and normal guinea-pigs of approximately equal size were stunned and then killed by exsanguination. The blood was allowed to clot at room temperature for 20 minutes, centrifuged at 0°, and the serum removed. The C2 and C4 content of these sera were then estimated by the haemolytic assay. Materials obtained from two homozygous, two heterozygous C4-deficient, and four normal guinea-pigs were examined. In each case, the results were based on at least duplicate, and in some cases triplicate, cultures of the cell and tissue preparations. Peritoneal exudates (PE) were induced by injecting approximately 7 ml of a 3 per cent starch suspension intraperitoneally into normal, heterozygous and homozygous C4-deficient guinea-pigs 72 hours before harvesting the exudate. The PE cells were collected in Hanks's balanced salt solution containing heparin 10 μ/ml, washed three times at 10° in medium 199 (Microbiological Associates, Bethesda, Maryland) containing penicillin 50 μ/ml and streptomycin 50 ug/ml (M199) and transferred to 35 × 10 mm Petri dishes (Falcon Plastics, Los Angeles, California). They were cultured in M199 supplemented with 10 per cent heated (2 hours at 56°) foetal calf serum (Grand Island Biological Company, Grand Island, New York) (M199 FCS) for 2 hours at 37° in a humidified 5 per cent CO_2, 95 per cent air atmosphere. After this period of incubation, the dishes were washed four times with M199 at room temperature to remove non-adherent PE cells, and then 2.0 ml of either M199 FCS or Neuman and Tytell's (N/T) serumless medium (Grand Island Biological Company) were added to the monolayers. In addition, the liver and spleen of each of the animals were removed and placed immediately in M199 at 0°. The tissues were minced, washed three times in M199 and then incubated for 1 hour at 0° to permit release of preformed C2 and C4, then washed

163

once again in cold M199. Measured portions (35–50 mg) of minced tissues were then transferred to 30-ml plastic tissue culture flasks (Falcon Plastics) and incubated in 3·5 ml of M199 FCS.

The capacity of tissues isolated from affected and normal guinea-pigs to incorporate ^{14}C-labelled amino acids into C4 protein was examined by a method already described in detail (Colten, 1971). Briefly, measured portions of liver and spleen fragments were each incubated at 37° or at 4° in M199 FCS in which ^{14}C-labelled leucine, isoleucine, lysine, and valine (New England Nuclear Corporation, Boston, Massachusetts) final concentration 1 μCi/ml) were substituted for the corresponding unlabelled amino acids. After 72 hours, the media were removed, dialysed, and then concentrated approximately 15-fold. The samples were then mixed with an equal volume of normal guinea-pig serum and placed in wells cut in 1 per cent agarose opposite guinea-pig anti-guinea-pig C4 antiserum.* Forty-eight hours later, the immunodiffusion plates were washed, dried, and radiolabelling of the precipitin lines detected by exposing the plates to Kodak X-ray film for 6 weeks.

Incorporation of ^{14}C-labelled amino acids by the tissues into total nondialysable cell products was detected by dissolving 20 μl of the concentrated dialysed media in 10 ml of Aquasol® (New England Nuclear Corporation) scintillation fluid and counting for 1 minute in a Packard Tri-Carb liquid scintillation spectrometer.

Heat-killed pneumococci type II were kindly supplied by Dr Erwin Gelfand.

RESULTS

C2 AND C4 CONTENT IN SERUM OF C4-DEFICIENT AND NORMAL GUINEA-PIGS

The results of haemolytic titrations of C2 and C4 in the sera of heterozygous and homozygous C4-deficient, and normal guinea-pigs, summarized in Table 1, show that the heterozygous deficient animal had approximately 45 per cent of the normal C4 level and 75 per cent of the normal C2 level. No C4 was detectable in the serum of the homozygous deficient animal, and the C2 content was about 30 per cent of normal. These results are comparable to previously published values for C2 and C4 in the sera of C4-deficient guinea-pigs (Frank *et al.*, 1971).

C4 SYNTHESIS BY ISOLATED LIVER AND SPLEEN

The *in vitro* synthesis of C4 by isolated fragments of liver and spleen was studied by incubating the tissues in M199 FCS at 37° and at 4°. At timed intervals, aliquots of the tissue culture media were removed, immediately diluted in ice-cold VBS-sucrose buffer, and assayed for haemolytically active C4. In this and subsequent experiments, the average rates of C4 and/or C2 synthesis were calculated from the amount of complement produced over the first 16–18 hours in culture. After 18–20 hours, the rates of synthesis in all primary cultures declined significantly, presumably due to limiting factors in tissue culture. The results listed in Table 2 indicate that the rate of C4 production by liver isolated from the heterozygous deficient animal was approximately 42 per cent of normal and that no significant C4 synthesis by homozygous deficient liver or spleen was detected. The serum of the heterozygous deficient animal from which the tissues were obtained had 44 per cent of the normal C4 content.

* The anti-C4 antiserum was prepared as previously described (Frank *et al.*, 1971).

Starch-induced peritoneal exudate cells from another set of affected and normal guinea-pigs were isolated and tested for their capacity to produce C4 *in vitro*. The results of this experiment shown in Fig. 1 indicate that the relative amounts of C4 produced by cells obtained from homozygous and heterozygous deficient animals were similar to the relative serum concentrations of C4; i.e. C4 production *in vitro* by heterozygous deficient cells was approximately 30 per cent of normal, and the serum concentration about 37 per cent of normal.

TABLE 1

HAEMOLYTICALLY ACTIVE C2 AND C4 IN THE SERA OF HOMOZYGOUS AND HETEROZYGOUS C4-DEFICIENT AND NORMAL GUINEA-PIGS

Guinea-Pig	C4		C2	
	Titre*	Ratio Affected/normal	Titre*	Ratio Affected/normal
Homozygous C4-deficient	<5	$<6.6 \times 10^{-6}$	19,300	0·30
Heterozygous C4-deficient	332,000	0·44	48,300	0·73
Normal	745,000	—	66,000	—

* Dilution of serum yielding 63 per cent lysis (average of one effective molecule per indicator cell).

TABLE 2

RATE OF C4 SYNTHESIS *in vitro* BY TISSUES FROM HOMOZYGOUS AND HETEROZYGOUS C4-DEFICIENT AND NORMAL GUINEA-PIGS

Tissue	Source of Tissue	C4 effective molecules ($\times 10^{-8}$) per 100 mg tissue per hour	Ratio Affected/normal
Liver	Homozygous	0·02*	0·003
	Heterozygous	2·8	0·42
	Normal	6·7	–
Spleen	Homozygous	0·2*	0·008
	Normal	25·0	–

* Not significantly different from rate of C4 production by tissues maintained at 4°.

C2 SYNTHESIS BY ISOLATED PE CELLS

In these experiments, PE cells (1.2×10^6/dish) isolated from a homozygous C4-deficient and a normal guinea-pig were incubated in N/T medium and in N/T medium containing approximately 300 heat-killed pneumococci per PE cell.[1] At timed intervals, aliquots were removed, assayed for C2 and C4 content, and the rates of C2 and C4 production were calculated. The results are summarized in Table 3. Again, no C4 production by homozygous deficient cells was detectable. C2 production in unstimulated cultures of homozygous deficient cells was 46 per cent of normal. In the same animal, the serum C2 content

[1]Pneumococci were utilized as a stimulant of complement biosynthesis since preliminary experiments showed that phagocytosis of certain particles by normal macrophages led to a 3–8-fold increase in the rates of C2 and C4 production (Colten, unpublished observations).

was 37 per cent of normal. In cultures exposed to heat-killed pneumococci, the rate of C2 synthesis by each cell preparation was increased. The increase in rate of C2 synthesis by 'deficient' cells, however, was proportionately greater than normal so that in stimulated cultures homozygous deficient cells were producing C2 at approximately the same rate as normal.

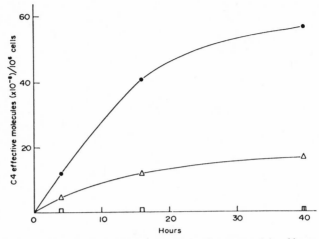

Fig. 1. Production of C4 *in vitro* by PE cells collected from homozygous (□) and heterozygous (△) C4-deficient and normal (●) guinea-pigs. The proportion of large mononuclear cells in each preparation was approximately 65 per cent. PE cells from affected and normal guinea-pigs could not be distinguished morphologically. Serum C4 content of normal guinea-pig, $1·16 \times 10^{14}$ effective molecules/ml; of heterozygous C4-deficient, $4·29 \times 10^{13}$ effective molecules/ml (37 per cent of normal); and of homozygous C4-deficient, less than $7·5 \times 10^7$ effective molecules/ml (less than 0·0006 per cent normal).

TABLE 3

RATE OF C2 AND C4 SYNTHESIS *in vitro* BY PERITONEAL EXUDATE (PE) CELLS FROM C4-DEFICIENT AND NORMAL GUINEA-PIGS

Source of PE	Heat-killed pneumococci added to culture	Effective molecules ($\times 10^{-8}$)/10^6 cells/hour	
		C2	C4
Homozygous-deficient	—	0·30	0·0
Normal	—	0·65	1·3
Ratio: deficient/normal	—	0·46	—
Homozygous-deficient	+	1·50	0·0
Normal	+	1·64	3·4
Ratio: deficient/normal	+	0·93	—

The possibility was considered that C4-deficient serum might contain factors which affect the biosynthesis or stability of C2 and C4 or that some other factor operating *in vivo* might inhibit C2 and C4 production by cells and tissues from affected animals. The following experiments suggested that these possibilities were unlikely.

EFFECT OF C4-DEFICIENT AND NORMAL GUINEA-PIG SERUM ON THE *in vitro*
SYNTHESIS OF C2 AND C4 BY NORMAL PE CELLS

Serum from a normal guinea-pig and from a C4-deficient animal were inactivated at 56
for 2 hours. Normal PE cells (1.5×10^6/dish) were incubated at 37° in N/T medium alone
or in medium containing the heat inactivated C4-deficient (1/100) or normal guinea-pig
serum (1/100). At timed intervals, aliquots of the media were removed, assayed for C2
and C4 activity, and the rates of C2 and C4 production were calculated. The results in
Table 4 show that addition of either normal or C4-deficient serum to the cultures resulted
in a 5–6-fold increase in the rate of synthesis of C2 and C4. Furthermore, there was no
significant difference in the capacity of normal and deficient serum to stimulate C2 and C4
synthesis.

TABLE 4

EFFECT OF NORMAL AND C4-DEFICIENT GUINEA-PIG SERUM ON THE RATE OF SYNTHESIS OF C2 AND C4
BY NORMAL GUINEA-PIG PE CELLS

PE in medium containing	C2 effective molecules ($\times 10^{-8}$) per 10^6 cells per hour	C4 effective molecules ($\times 10^{-8}$) per 10^6 cells per hour
C4-deficient serum	1·6	2·15
Normal serum	1·7	2·46
No supplement	0·27	0·39

* Sera heated 56° for 2 hours, then each used at a dilution of 1/100 in Neuman and Tytell medium.

TABLE 5

BIOSYNTHESIS OF C2 AND C4 BY GUINEA-PIG PERITONEAL EXUDATE (PE) CELLS
MAINTAINED IN TISSUE CULTURE

Source of PE	Time *in vitro* (weeks)				
	0·5	2	3	4	5
	C2 effective molecules ($\times 10^{-8}$)*/culture				
C4-deficient†	21·6	19·5	16·2	20·7	50·5
Normal	46·9	47·7	40·5	55·5	110·0
Deficient/Normal	0·46	0·41	0·40	0·37	0·46
	C4 effective molecules ($\times 10^{-8}$)*/culture Time *in vitro* (weeks)				
C4-deficient†	0·0	0·0	0·0	0·0	ND
Normal	93·6	18·0	9·3	16·2	ND
Deficient/Normal	—	—	—	—	—

* C2 and C4 measured 48 hours after each medium change.
† Homozygous C4-deficient.

LONG-TERM PRODUCTION OF C2 AND C4 *in vitro*

Long-term primary cultures of PE cells from normal and homozygous deficient animals
were established and maintained in M199 FCS. The medium was changed weekly, and
48 hours after each medium change the C2 and C4 content of the tissue culture media
were determined. As shown in Table 5, the relative amounts of C2 and C4 produced by
cells from normal and deficient animals remained approximately constant over 4 weeks
in culture. The ratio of deficient/normal production of C2 was constant at about 0·40, and
there was no C4 production by deficient cells during this period, even though normal cells
continued to produce C4 up to 4 weeks after isolation *in vitro*.

167

The results of these experiments shown in Fig. 2 and Table 6 indicate that normal and C4-deficient tissues were equally capable of incorporating ^{14}C-labelled amino acids into total non-dialysable cell products and that this incorporation was highly temperature dependent (Table 6). In contrast, although normal guinea-pig spleen and liver incubated

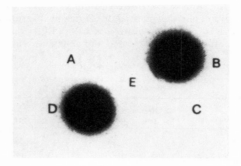

Fig. 2. *In vitro* incorporation of ^{14}C-labelled amino acids into C4 protein by guinea-pig spleen: radioimmunodiffusion of dialysed concentration tissue culture media. A, normal spleen at 4°; B, normal spleen at 37°; C, C4-deficient spleen at 4°; D, C4-deficient spleen at 37°; E, guinea-pig anti-C4 antiserum. Radiolabelled line between wells B + E corresponded exactly to precipitin line.

TABLE 6

IN VITRO INCORPORATION OF ^{14}C-LABELLED AMINO ACIDS INTO NON-DIALYSABLE CELL PRODUCTS BY GUINEA-PIG TISSUES

Tissue	Guinea-pig	Temperature (°)	CPM*
Liver	C4-deficient	37	4560
Liver	Normal	37	3640
Liver	C4-deficient	4	240
Liver	Normal	4	220
Spleen	C4-deficient	37	16110
Spleen	Normal	37	15860
Spleen	C4-deficient	4	180
Spleen	Normal	4	360

* Counts per minute in 20-μl sample of dialysed concentrated tissue culture media.

at 37° were capable of incorporating the radiolabelled amino acids into specific protein, immunochemically identified as C4, no labelling of C4 by homozygous C4-deficient tissues could be demonstrated. Fig. 2, the radioautograph of an immunoprecipitin analysis of radiolabelled C4, showed incorporation of ^{14}C-amino acids by normal guinea-pig spleen but not by C4-deficient spleen. Incorporation of radiolabelled amino acids by normal and C4-deficient liver into total protein was significantly less than incorporation by spleen (Table 6). As a consequence, only a faint radiolabelled C4 precipitin line was detected

168

between guinea-pig anti-C4 antiserum and medium from the normal liver culture. No radiolabelled C4 was detected in medium from C4-deficient liver cultures.

DISCUSSION

Recent technical developments have made it possible to study in tissue culture some of the factors that govern the rate of complement biosynthesis. We have applied these methods to an investigation of a genetically controlled abnormality of complement production (C4 deficiency). This autosomal recessive trait is of particular interest for several reasons: (1) it has been shown that both C2 (Rubin, Borsos, Rapp and Colten, 1972) and C4 (Littleton, Kessler and Burkholder, 1970) are produced by large mononuclear cells (macrophages) and that, at least in some cases, individual cells capable of synthesizing C2 are also synthesizing C4 (Wyatt, Colten and Borsos, 1971); (2) it is known that most guinea-pigs deficient in C4 have a moderate reduction in serum C2 content (Frank *et al.*, 1971), therefore, it is possible to study C2 and C4 biosynthesis using a single affected animal; and (3) these studies provide a model for the investigation of other abnormalities of complement production in man and experimental animals.

The results of these experiments showed that tissues and cells isolated from homozygous C4-deficient animals and maintained in culture for prolonged periods were incapable of synthesizing C4. Furthermore, there was no evidence that reduced output of C4 by these cells was a consequence of secretory block, i.e. intracellular C4 content was low or absent in cells isolated from C4-deficient animals. As predicted, cells from heterozygous deficient animals produced C4 at a rate intermediate between the normal and homozygous animals. The observation that this abnormality of C4 production persisted in culture up to 4 weeks after isolation of the cells *in vitro* indicates that the abnormality is probably not the result of factors *in vivo* which might secondarily affect the rate of C4 production. It is interesting to note, however, that normal cells maintained in long-term culture produced C4 at only about 12 per cent the rate observed in freshly isolated cells. At the present time, we have no explanation for this observation, but it is possible that a factor or factors *in vivo* increase the rate of C4 production by normal cells. Support for this possibility is given by experiments which show about a 6-fold increase in the rate of C4 production by heated (56°, 2 hours) normal or C4-deficient guinea-pig serum; i.e. serum may contain a heat-stable factor which accelerates the rate of C4 synthesis. Attempts to identify this factor are now in progress.

The studies of C2 production by C4-deficient cells in culture also demonstrated an abnormality of C2 synthesis. The rates of C2 and C4 synthesis, however, appeared to be under separate control since stimulation of C4-deficient PE cells in culture led to an increase in the rate of C2 biosynthesis with no measurable effect on C4 production. Furthermore, although homozygous C4-deficient animals all have a total deficiency of C4, most, but not all, have significantly reduced C2 levels. Studies now in progress, using somatic hybrids of C4-deficient PE cells with human cells, should make it possible to identify more precisely the details of these biochemical abnormalities of C2 and C4 production.

REFERENCES

ALPER, C. A., PROPP, R. P., KLEMPERER, M. R. and ROSEN, F. S. (1969). 'Inherited deficiency of the third component of complement (C'3).' *J. clin. Invest.*, **48**, 553.

COLTEN, H. R. (1972) 'Ontogeny of the human complement system: *In vitro* biosynthesis of individual complement components by fetal tissues.' *J. clin. Invest.* (In press).

COLTEN, H. R. and WYATT, H. V. (1971). 'Biosynthesis of serum complement.' In *Proceedings of the V International Symposium on Biological Activities of Complement.* S. Karger, Basel, (in press).

DONALDSON, V. H. and EVANS, P. R. (1963). 'A biochemical abnormality in hereditary angioneurotic edema.' *Amer. J. Med.*, **35**, 37.

ELLMAN, L., GREEN, I., and FRANK, M. M. (1970). 'Genetically controlled total deficiency of the fourth component of complement in the guinea pig.' *Science*, **170**, 74.

FRANK, M. M., MAY, J., GAITHER, T., and ELLMAN, L. (1971). '*In vitro* studies of complement function in sera of C4-deficient guinea pigs.' *J. exp. Med.*, **134**, 176.

KLEMPERER, M. R., WOODWORTH, H. C., ROSEN, F. S. and AUSTEN, K. F. (1966). 'Hereditary deficiency of the second component of complement(C'2) in man.' *J. clin. Invest.*, **45**, 880.

LITTLETON, C., KESSLER, D. and BURKHOLDER, P. M. (1970). 'Cellular basis for synthesis of the fourth component of guinea-pig complement as determined by a haemolytic plaque technique.' *Immunology*, **18**, 691.

OPFERKUCH, W., RAPP, H. J., COLTEN, H. R. and BORSOS, T. (1971). 'Immune hemolysis and the functional properties of the second (C2) and fourth (C4) components of complement. III. The hemolytic efficiency of human and guinea pig C2 and C4.' *J. Immunol.*, **106**, 927.

RAPP, H. J. and BORSOS, T. (1970.) 'Molecular Basis of Complement Action.' Appleton-Century-Crofts, New York, New York.

Rosenberg, L. T. and Tachibana, D. F. (1962). 'Activity of mouse complement.' *J. Immunol.*, **89**, 861.

ROTHER, K. O., ROTHER, U., MÜLLER-EBERHARD, H. J. and NILSSON, U. R. (1966). 'Deficiency of the sixth component of complement in rabbits with an inherited complement defect.' *J. exp. Med.*, **124**, 773.

RUBIN, D. J., BORSOS, T., RAPP, H. J. and COLTEN, H. R. (1971). 'Synthesis of the second component of guinea pig complement *in vitro*.' *J. Immunol.*, **106**, 295.

WYATT, H. V., COLTEN, H. R. and BORSOS, T. (1971). 'Production of the second (C2) and fourth (C4) components of guinea pig complement by single peritoneal exudate cells: Evidence that one cell may produce both components.' *Fed. Proc.*, **30**, 355.

AUTHOR INDEX

Agnello, V., 146
Alper, Chester A., 154
Arroyave, Carlos M., 85

Bing, David H., 32, 45
Borsos, Tibor, 58
Butler, William T., 116

Colten, Harvey R., 58, 154, 162

de Bracco, M.M.E., 146

Frank, M.M., 162

Hoffmann, Louis G., 100

Kunkel, H.G., 146

Müller-Eberhard, Hans J., 85

Niedermeier, William, 116
Nilsson, U.R., 66

Rapp, Herbert J., 58

Sassano, Felix G., 58
Shelton, Emma, 137
Sledge, Carlos R., 32
Stroud, Robert M., 10, 116, 123, 137

Taylor, F.B., Jr., 66
Thompson, James J., 100
Tomar, R.H., 66

Yonemasu, Kunio, 10, 116, 123, 137

KEY-WORD TITLE INDEX